Pre-Hospital Aı
Handbook

CH00730311

Tim Lowes • Amy Gospel
Andrew Griffiths • Jeremy Henning

Pre-Hospital Anesthesia Handbook

Second Edition

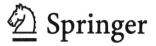 Springer

Tim Lowes
Intensive Care Unit
James Cook University Hospital
Middlesbrough
UK

Amy Gospel
Tyne and Wear
UK

Andrew Griffiths
The York Hospital
Middlesbrough
UK

Jeremy Henning
James Cook University Hospital
Middlesbrough
UK

ISBN 978-3-319-23089-4   ISBN 978-3-319-23090-0   (eBook)
DOI 10.1007/978-3-319-23090-0

Library of Congress Control Number: 2015958249

Springer Cham Heidelberg New York Dordrecht London

Printed on acid-free paper

Springer International Publishing AG Switzerland is part of Springer Science+Business Media (www.springer.com)

Foreword

The dramatic changes in the management of critically ill or injured patients in the pre-hospital environment that follow the implementation of lessons learnt in austere distant zones precede the publication of focused, evidence-based guides and manuals. This manual is therefore a great step forwards in training and assessment.

The commitment expressed in the Darzi report (High Quality Care for All – NHS Next Stage Review Final Report 2008) to provide the best care for all patients does mean that there will be occasions when primary resuscitation of patients is followed by a more prolonged transfer to definitive care. The opportunities to start and continue critical care of seriously ill patients by skilled anesthetists should provide the same benefits for civilian populations as has been demonstrated in hostile operations; a clear message from the Healthcare Commission (2009).

The authors are all experts in both the practical clinical application and the academic and research aspects of pre-hospital care. This manual covers the most important aspects of anesthesia and rightly concentrates on the safe and rapid establishment of a secure airway as part of the ongoing care of the patient. The techniques for rapid sequence induction of anesthesia are discussed and just as importantly so are the necessary subsequent anesthesia and sedation techniques.

This manual should be essential reading for all involved in the pre-hospital arena from paramedical to medical staff. It is a model for others to follow and it is a privilege to be asked to write this foreword.

Professor David Lockey
Consultant in Intensive Care Medicine
and Anaesthesia, North Bristol NHS Trust
Honorary Professor of Trauma
and Pre-hospital Medicine, Bristol University
Clinical Director, Severn Major Trauma Network
Research and Development Lead,
London's Air Ambulance, Vice Chairman,
Faculty of Pre-hospital,Royal College
of Surgeons of Edinburgh

Preface to the Second Edition

Since the publication of the first edition, Pre-Hospital Emergency Medicine (PHEM) has evolved significantly. In the UK there are over twenty helicopter-based air ambulance services and where previously many of these only had paramedic crews, the majority now deploy with a combined physician and paramedic crew.

There are now many Consultants in Anaesthesia or Emergency Medicine who have a regular air ambulance day within their job plan. These Consultants are expected to have at least a 50 % commitment to their base specialty, so at least 700 will be required nationally to support the current services. When the first edition was published, PHEM training was variable and dependent on individuals and local systems. PHEM has now been formally approved by the UK General Medical Council (GMC) as a medical sub-specialty of the existing specialties of Emergency Medicine, Anaesthetics, Intensive Care and Acute Medicine. Therefore, an increasing number of the physicians on board will be doctors undertaking formal PHEM training.

A key part of PHEM training is the provision of anaesthesia in the pre-hospital environment. The Great North Air Ambulance Service (GNAAS) Pre-hospital Anaesthesia (PHA) 2-day course has continued to receive excellent feedback from the many doctors and paramedics who have filled every course to date. The PHA Handbook covers all aspects of PHA, and the second edition includes changes in practice and additional published evidence from the last five years. An important element in the safe and successful practice of PHA is Crew Resource Management (CRM) and a whole new chapter reflects the importance of this.

GNAAS continues to be funded by public charitable donation to provide both aircraft and medical staff. The authors will continue to donate all royalties from the sale of this book to the charity fund, specifically in order to improve the equipment required to maintain the high standard of training, both on the course and undertaken on a regular basis by the crew.

Middlesbrough and York, UK   Tim Lowes
                                                    Amy Gospel
                                                    Andy Griffiths
                                                    Jeremy Henning

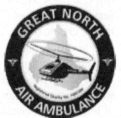

Preface to the First Edition

Over the past few years in the United Kingdom there have been many reports into trauma which have highlighted poor pre-hospital care as a major cause of possibly preventable deaths. Similar issues have been identified internationally. Many pre-hospital systems have therefore developed standard operating procedures that involve inducing anesthesia for airway control.

Many physician providers find it difficult to access training in this area, and assisting anesthesia is outside most paramedics' curriculum. This was a problem we faced at the Great North Air Ambulance Service. To address this, we developed a two day course to provide an introduction to pre-hospital anesthetic practice. This book has evolved from the manual we wrote for the course, which we continue to run three times a year.

It is clear that pre-hospital anesthesia remains a controversial procedure, with many conflicting papers written about its benefits and risks. For this reason, anyone undertaking it has a duty to ensure they undertake it safely and within a well governed system. A book cannot provide clinical experience, however, we hope that it will give a good knowledge-base to guide and develop practice. The available evidence is discussed, relevant pharmacology is explained and a system to provide pre-hospital anesthesia is presented.

We hope this book will prove to be an enjoyable read that will encourage many to develop their pre-hospital anesthetic practice. It has to be the hope of all working in this world that no patient ever dies from having inadequate airway control before their admission to hospital.

The authors acknowledge the support that the Great North Air Ambulance Service has given in the evolution of the course, and are donating all of their royalties from the sales of this book to the charity fund.

Middlesbrough, UK   Andy Griffiths
                                                  Tim Lowes
                                           Jeremy Henning

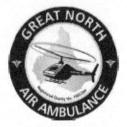

Aims and Objectives

- To be aware of the risks and benefits of Pre-hospital Anaesthesia (PHA)
- To understand and be able to apply the concepts of Crew Resource Management (CRM)
- To be familiar with the equipment and monitoring required to safely undertake Pre-hospital Rapid Sequence Intubation (PRSI)
- To increase competence at managing PRSI, including failed intubation
- To develop a comprehensive knowledge of the pharmacology of all PHA drugs, including indications, contraindications, doses and side effects
- To gain confidence in the preparation and transfer of the intubated patient and management of potential adverse events during transfer

Note: This handbook assumes experience with intubation, simple airway manoeuvres, bag-valve-mask ventilation and Advanced Life Support/Advanced Trauma Life Support protocols.

Contents

List of Authors

Col. Tim Lowes, MBBS, FRCA, FICM, Dip IMC.RCS(Ed), L/RAMC
Consultant in Anaesthesia & Intensive Care
James Cook University Hospital, Middlesbrough, UK

Military Clinical Director
Defence Medical Group (North), UK

Dr. Amy Gospel, MBBS, BMed Sci(Hons), FRCA, Dip IMC.RCS(Ed)
Anaesthetic & Pre-Hospital Emergency Medicine Registrar, Health Education North-East/Great North Air Ambulance Service/North East Ambulance Service, UK

Col. Andrew Griffiths, OBE, MBBS, BMed Sci, FRCA, CMgr MCMI, L/RAMC
Consultant in Anaesthesia, The York Hospital, York, UK

Col. Jeremy Henning, MBBS, FICM, FRCA, L/RAMC
Consultant in Anaesthesia & Intensive Care,
James Cook University Hospital, Middlesbrough, UK

Abbreviations

AAGBI	Association of Anaesthetists of Great Britain and Ireland
ACCS	Acute care common stem
ACoT	Acute coagulopathy of trauma
ALS	Advanced life support
ARDS	Acute respiratory distress syndrome
ASA	American Society of Anesthesiologists
BMI	Body mass index
BP	Blood pressure
BURP	Backward upward rightward pressure
BVM	Bag-valve-mask
CBRN	Chemical, biological, radiological, nuclear
COPD	Chronic obstructive pulmonary disease
CPAP	Continuous positive airway pressure
CPP	Cerebral perfusion pressure
CRM	Crew resource management
ECG	Electrocardiogram
ED	Emergency department
EM	Emergency medicine
EMS	Emergency medical service
$ETCO_2$	End-tidal carbon dioxide
ETT	Endotracheal tube
FiO_2	Fraction of inspired oxygen
GCS	Glasgow coma score
GP	General practitioner
HEMS	Helicopter emergency medical service
HMEF	Heat moisture exchange filter
IBTPHEM	Intercollegiate board for training in pre-hospital emergency medicine
ICP	Intracranial pressure

ICU	Intensive care unit
I:E	Inspiratory:expiratory
IM	Intramuscular
IO	Intraosseous
IV	Intravenous
LMA	Laryngeal mask airway
MAP	Mean arterial pressure
MERIT	Medical emergency response incident team
MERT	Medical emergency response team
MILS	Manual in-line stabilisation
M&M	Morbidity and mortality
NIBP	Non-invasive blood pressure
NMBA	Neuromuscular blocking agents
NPA	Nasopharyngeal airway
OPA	Oropharyngeal airway
$PaCO_2$	Partial pressure of CO_2 in arterial blood
PaO_2	Partial pressure of O_2 in arterial blood
PALM	Pharmacologically assisted LMA
PCI	Percutaneous coronary intervention
PEA	Pulseless electrical activity
PEEP	Positive end expiratory pressure
PHA	Pre-hospital anaesthesia
PHEM	Pre-hospital emergency medicine
PRF	Patient report form
PRSI	Pre-hospital rapid sequence intubation
RCT	Randomised controlled trial
RSI	Rapid sequence induction/intubation
RTC	Road traffic collision
SAD	Supraglottic airway device
SBP	Systolic blood pressure
SOP	Standard operating procedure
SpO_2	Oxygen saturation
TBI	Traumatic brain injury
TCA	Traumatic cardiac arrest
TRM	Team resource management
TXA	Tranexamic acid
UK	United Kingdom
US	United States
VF	Ventricular fibrillation

Chapter 1
Introduction

By the end of this chapter you will be able to:

- Understand the term "rapid sequence induction"
- Discuss the evidence regarding who should perform rapid sequence induction
- Understand the challenges of pre-hospital anaesthesia
- Discuss the evidence for and against pre-hospital anaesthesia

1.1 Pre-hospital Anaesthesia (PHA)

Emergency anaesthesia, intubation and ventilation are often key interventions in the management of the seriously unwell or injured patient. Indications for such intervention encompass a wide range of pathologies including; airway compromise, respiratory insufficiency, reduced consciousness, and requirement for sedation/anaesthesia to enable other care. These are discussed further in Chap. 2.

Emergency anaesthesia most commonly takes place in operating theatres, critical care units, and hospital emergency departments. There is, however, a group of patients in whom indications for emergency anaesthesia are present prior to hospital arrival. Commencing this intervention earlier in their care pathway, in the pre-hospital phase rather than awaiting hospital arrival, should improve their outcome.

T. Lowes et al., *Pre-Hospital Anesthesia Handbook*,
DOI 10.1007/978-3-319-23090-0_1,
© Springer-Verlag London 2016

This handbook includes the evidence, indications, contra-indications, preparation and performance of pre-hospital anaesthesia (PHA). It also covers the equally important subject of post-intubation management, including the Prevention and management of adverse events during transfer. Other techniques usually classed under the remit of anaesthesia, including sedation and analgesia will also be covered, but the main focus remains PHA.

1.2   Rapid Sequence Intubation (RSI)

The vast majority of emergency anaesthetics undertaken in the pre-hospital environment will be commenced with an anaesthetic technique based on a rapid sequence induction with tracheal intubation. Rapid sequence induction is used to induce anaesthesia and to ensure optimal intubating conditions in as short a time as possible (Box 1.1). 'Rapid sequence induction' is therefore synonymous with 'rapid sequence intubation'.

Box 1.1: Aims of RSI
- Rapidly induce anaesthesia[a]
- Rapidly achieve complete muscle relaxation to provide optimum intubating conditions
- Prevent airway soiling

[a]In unconscious patients, the aim of the induction drug(s) is to attenuate the physiological response to intubation (i.e., hypertension, tachycardia and raised intracranial pressure).

RSI is used in emergency anaesthesia to protect the airway from soiling by oral contaminants (e.g. blood) or regurgitated stomach content. It is also utilised in the management of critically ill patients with pathologies such as acute lung injury or bronchospasm, where mask ventilation may be insufficient to generate the necessary pressures to maintain adequate oxygenation. Prompt intubation should minimise the period of potential hypoxia by immediately providing the ability to achieve increased airway pressures and positive end expiratory pressure (PEEP).

RSI was originally described as a sequence of 15 steps by Stept and Safar (1970). Sellick's landmark publication on cricoid pressure in 1961 (Sellick 1961) had already alluded to the benefits of preoxygenation, intravenous barbiturate and a short-acting muscle relaxant as the ideal technique when there was risk of regurgitation on induction. RSI removed the requirement to ventilate with a face mask, and therefore mitigated the associated risks of gastric insufflation and subsequent regurgitation prior to intubation. The primary aim of RSI was to improve the safety of anaesthesia for emergency surgery, where the risk of aspiration is highest.

Contemporary pre-hospital RSI includes modifications to improve safety, practicality and reduce physiological disturbance. These include: the use of opioids and long-acting neuromuscular blocking agents, a low threshold for early release of cricoid pressure and techniques to improve oxygenation during RSI including nasal supplementation and even mask ventilation.

There are several pharmacological recipes used to achieve RSI, but all employ a combination of:

- An induction drug to provide amnesia and obtund the response to intubation e.g. Ketamine, Etomidate, or Propofol, ± additional agents to further obtund physiological responses e.g. Fentanyl or Alfentanil.
- A neuromuscular blocking drug to provide paralysis and optimum intubating conditions e.g. Rocuronium or Suxamethonium

1.2.1 Who Should Perform RSI?

Within hospital practice, emergency anaesthesia outside of the operating theatre commonly occurs in the emergency department (ED) and critical care areas. The conduct of RSI in these areas is associated with a higher rate of poor views at laryngoscopy and increased complication rates (Taryle et al. 1979). The fourth National Audit Project (NAP4) of the Royal College of Anaesthetists and the Difficult Airway Society established a 12 month registry of major complications of airway management across NHS hospitals in the UK (Cook et al. 2011). It found that at least one in four major airway complications reported, occurred in the Intensive Care Unit (ICU) or ED, and that the outcomes of these events were more likely to lead to permanent harm or death than events in operating theatres. Such findings may relate to the difficulties faced by staff working outside of the familiar theatre environment and with less familiar equipment. This problem is further compounded by the fact that the sub-set of patients requiring emergency airway interventions tend to be more physiologically compromised, have a higher requirement for manual in-line stabilisation (MILS), and are generally more complex to manage.

Historically, within the UK, anaesthetists have conducted almost all in-hospital emergency anaesthesia. As different specialties have developed, notably Emergency Medicine (EM) and Intensive Care Medicine (ICM), RSI is increasingly also undertaken by other clinicians. The curricula of the Faculty of Intensive Care Medicine (2014) and Royal College of Emergency Medicine (2010) both reflect this, with emergency anaesthesia and airway management being an essential part of training.

Whether non-anaesthetic staff should be performing RSI unsupervised by an anaesthetist as *routine* practice has been much debated, and significant variation in practices exists between different hospitals. Previous UK studies of ED RSI comparing EM staff to anaesthetists found that anaesthetists achieved significantly better views at laryngoscopy and had a greater success rate for first-pass intubations (Graham et al. 2003; Stevenson et al. 2007). A recent census of UK-wide ED airway management found that 80 % of ED RSIs were performed by anaesthetists, predominantly senior anaesthetic trainees of ST3 and above (Benger and Hopkinson 2011).

In contrast, a recent study published by Edinburgh Royal Infirmary, had EM physicians performing 78 % of intubations, and anaesthetists 22 %, utilising a joint RSI protocol, in which a senior anaesthetist provides immediate support whilst trained EM staff perform RSI (Kerslake et al. 2015). This study is one of the largest series reported, including 3738 ED intubations at one large Scottish teaching hospital. Over the 13 years reviewed (1999–2011) they found that EM physicians achieved similar views but lower initial intubation success rates for RSI when compared to anaesthetists. Overall intubation was successful in 99.6 % of patients, with first time successful tracheal intubation in 85 % (anaesthetists 92 %, EM consultants 94 % and EM trainees 83 %; $p < 0.001$). In subgroup analysis of intubations since 2007, the difference in initial success rate between ED and anaesthetic physicians is no longer apparent (87 % vs. 88 % respectively). One explanation could be that the intubation skills of EM physicians have improved due to increased training and skills maintenance in anaesthesia and emergency airway management. It may also demonstrate the advantages of collaboration between anaesthetists and ED staff in performing emergency airway management, with prediction of 'difficult' intubation and use of the most appropriately experienced physician for the initial intubation attempt. Complications occurred in 9.4 % of RSIs, with no significant difference in rate of complications between anaesthetists and EM physicians.

In a similar prospective study, RSIs performed by critical care staff, encompassing those taking place in the ED, ICU and wards, demonstrated that non-anaesthetists had a significantly higher incidence of unsuccessful intubation attempts and multiple attempts, compared with anaesthetists (10.8 % vs. 3.9 %) (Reid et al. 2004). However overall (albeit self-reported) complication rates were not significantly different between groups.

A large US study reinforces the importance of optimising the intubation conditions for RSI, by suggesting that the incidence of complications increases significantly when more than one attempt at intubation is required (Thomas 2004). This was replicated in the findings of Kerslake et al (2015), where complications occurred in 8 % of patients overall; however the incidence increased significantly with the number of intubation attempts (7 % with one attempt, 15 % with two attempts and 32 % with three attempts). Such complications include desaturation/hypoxia, hypotension, vomiting/regurgitation, arrhythmia, cardiac arrest, misplaced endotracheal tubes and airway trauma.

In their retrospective study of patients intubated within the first 2 h of arrival at a Level 1 trauma centre, Sise et al. (2009) found a similar significant correlation with the rate of complications increasing with the number of intubation attempts. They also demonstrated that complications were more common when resident physicians (postgraduate years 2–4) were involved in the intubation, than when more senior physicians took the first intubation attempt (14.2 % vs. 9.7 %), and that they were significantly less successful at first intubation attempt (78 % vs. 92 %). This unsurprising relationship between training level and intubation success, was also seen by Kerslake et al. (2015). EM consultants had intubation success comparable to anaesthetists; however EM trainees had significantly lower success rates.

In summary, intubation outside the theatre environment has less chance of first time success and more chance of complications. Current evidence demonstrates that, as one may expect by virtue of their training and continuing experience, anaesthetists are more likely to gain a better view at laryngoscopy and intubate successfully, with fewer complications. Physicians of other specialty backgrounds can achieve comparable intubation success, and it may be more appropriate for a senior EM physician to perform RSI than a junior anaesthetic trainee.

It should be remembered that familiarity with the side effects and appropriate doses of induction agents, along with the ability to minimise and manage adverse effects is as important as the ability to get the best view at laryngoscopy.

As with many things, the key factors in a safe and successful outcome, are appropriate training and ongoing maintenance of skills.

1.3   Pre-hospital RSI

1.3.1   The Pre-hospital Environment

The pre-hospital environment is one of the most challenging clinical settings in which to practice. It can be austere as well as emotionally and physically demanding. The conditions are at best suboptimal, characterised by difficult access to the patient, limited equipment, inclement weather conditions and poor lighting (too dark or too bright). All these factors and many other stressors can hinder the performance of an optimal pre-hospital RSI. The pre-hospital practitioner may also have less support in terms of additional medical assistance and specialist airway equipment in the event of difficulties. To compound matters, many patients will have sustained head or neck trauma, which may lead to a more challenging intubation, even in the controlled environment of a hospital (either directly e.g. airway blood/swelling or indirectly e.g. manual in-line stabilisation (MILS) of the neck. Despite these issues, the threshold to intubate is often lower. This can be influenced by the difficulties in managing a partially obstructed airway and/or an agitated patient during transfer to hospital, particularly if this is in a helicopter.

1.3.2   The Evidence for Pre-hospital RSI

Anecdotal reports suggest that pre-hospital RSI (PRSI) has been practised since the 1970s. The first report in the literature of drug-assisted pre-hospital intubation described paramedics using succinylcholine to assist intubation (Hedges et al. 1988). Over subsequent years, the technique has been progressively adapted from hospital practice.

Intubation and ventilation in hospital is considered a cornerstone in the management of critically ill patients. The optimum timing for this intervention has never been studied but it is assumed that the earlier the intervention takes place the greater the benefit it will offer. It has not been proven that RSI in the ED (vs. theatre or ICU) improves outcome and reduces mortality, and probably never will be, as it is now accepted practice. This has become the case with PRSI, although it is clearly possible that the risks of carrying out this procedure in the pre-hospital setting may outweigh the benefits in certain situations. In other words, when RSI is undertaken in suboptimal conditions there is the potential for increased morbidity and mortality. In the absence of appropriate personnel with the relevant training and equipment, a conservative approach may be appropriate.

Lossius et al. published a systematic literature review of pre-hospital intubation in 2011. They highlighted the difficulty in establishing an evidence-base for pre-hospital intubation when the available studies demonstrate such heterogeneity in procedures, providers, patients, systems and stated outcomes. In addition, the vast majority of publications are retrospective studies.

There is currently no randomised controlled data showing clear benefit in mortality or morbidity following pre-hospital intubation. The first randomised controlled trial of pre-hospital intubation involved paramedics intubating children without drugs (Gausche et al. 2000). In addition to the lack of physicians and drugs (i.e., not pre-hospital RSI), the study had major flaws.

The long-awaited 'Head Injury Retrieval Trial' (HIRT), which aimed to be the first prospective randomised controlled trial (RCT) evaluating the addition of pre-hospital physician care compared with paramedic only care for patients with severe head injury, has recently been published (Garner et al. 2015). Within the duration of the trial (2005–2011), changes in the ambulance service policies made physician treatment of these patients the expected standard of care, leading to significant protocol violation, non-compliance with recruitment and randomisation, and considerable crossover between groups. Using an 'as-treated' analysis of data, rather than the standard 'intention to treat' analysis, they were able to report a potential 30-day mortality reduction in adult patients with blunt trauma and Glasgow Coma Score (GCS) <9 receiving additional physician care, such as drug assisted intubation, but were not able to demonstrate a significant improvement in overall mortality or 6-month Glasgow Outcome Scores. Due to such potential bias in the study the findings are not conclusive; but it does highlight the difficulties in carrying out high-quality prospective pre-hospital research. It is suggested that future studies need to take place in settings where physician staffed teams are not part of the established standard care.

There have been numerous retrospective studies, and overall these have not provided clear evidence to support PHA either. Some of the studies suggest survival advantage (Winchell and Hoyt 1997; Arbabi et al. 2004). Others showed no improvement in neurological outcome or mortality (Stockinger and McSwain 2004). Other studies appeared to show an adverse outcome from pre-hospital intubation (Murray 2000; Eckstein et al. 2000).

The majority of studies are from the US (several from the same trauma database) and involved paramedics. Many used either no drugs or simply sedation with midazolam and no neuromuscular blocking drug. Both failed intubation and other complications are reduced by the use of neuromuscular blocking drugs (Bulger et al. 2005). These trials, most of which suggest inferior outcomes, are therefore clearly not applicable to pre-hospital RSI as currently practised by physician/paramedic pre-hospital teams. The study by Davis et al. of paramedic RSI in traumatic brain injury compared to historical controls was associated with an increase in mortality (Davis et al. 2003). Periods of reduced SpO_2, and hyperventilation were noted and the relatively limited training and experience of paramedics were cited as potentially important factors. These critical factors *are* still relevant today.

Services such as the Whatcom Medic One (Washington state) had a relatively small number of well-trained paramedics using a recognised pre-hospital RSI technique and reported very good results (Wang et al. 2004). It is perhaps not surprising that those with large numbers of paramedics with very limited training and only occasional RSI experience tended to show worse outcomes. Improved outcome has been demonstrated for patients transferred by helicopter compared to land ambulance (Davis et al. 2005). This may be due to speed of transfer to hospital, better trained staff or a combination of both.

Together this leads to the conclusion that small teams of well-trained staff on board helicopters are likely to improve outcomes if they are able to safely perform pre-hospital RSI for appropriate patients.

One way to respond to the studies available is to follow the principle of "Primum non nocere" (first, do no harm). Where clear evidence does not exist to demonstrate benefit, it may seem reasonable to assume that the minimum input to achieve a patent airway and adequate ventilation should be recommended. This can be achieved, in some cases by simple airway manoeuvres with or without the use of adjuncts and a bag-valve-mask. Although this does not confer any degree of airway protection, it may allow rapid transfer from the scene. Recognising a problem and doing simple manoeuvres well, *does* save lives.

There is an alternative view endorsed by the Great North Air Ambulance Service, the London Helicopter Emergency Medical Service (HEMS) and now many other physician-led pre-hospital medical services in the UK. It is a view that is based on the principle that optimal critical care provision should be available for those patients who require it at the earliest opportunity. In hospital this would invariably include intubation, and therefore pre-hospital anaesthesia is an essential part of HEMS training. Many helicopter systems worldwide now also deliver this capability as part of their service provision.

1.3.3   Is There a Need for PHA?

Current UK ambulance service airway management consists of a stepwise approach to airway management. Guidelines progress through: airway manoeuvres, airway adjuncts, supraglottic airway devices (SAD) (e.g. laryngeal mask airway (LMA) or I-gel®), and potentially tracheal intubation (if appropriately trained) in order to adequately maintain the airway (JRCALC 2013). Significant airway compromise is relatively uncommon in routine paramedic practice, and as a result most paramedics rarely perform advanced airway interventions unless they are operating as part of enhanced care teams. The lack of benefit and considerable complications associated with tracheal intubation without drugs, led to the 2008 recommendation that tracheal intubation should not be mandatory training for UK paramedics (Deakin et al. 2008). Many organisations, therefore, do not teach paramedics to intubate, although a number of paramedics do retain this skill.

At a similar time, deficiencies within pre-hospital airway management in the UK were highlighted by the 2007 National Confidential Enquiry into Patient Outcome and Death (NCEPOD) report 'Trauma – who cares' (NCEPOD 2007). It reported that 12.6 % of major trauma patients arrived in the emergency department with a partially or completely occluded airway, and these patients had a higher mortality. The principle recommendations of NCEPOD included the following statement, which has supported the increased provision of PHA across the UK:

> There is a high incidence of patients arriving at hospital with a partially or completely obstructed airway. Change is urgently required to provide a system that reliably provides a clear airway with good oxygenation and control of ventilation. This may be through the provision of personnel with the ability to provide anaesthesia and intubation in the pre-hospital phase… (NCEPOD 2007)

Recently a prospective observational study conducted in London 2012–2013 aimed to document the frequency of airway compromise in trauma patients in the pre-hospital phase of their care, and the need for advanced airway interventions (Lockey et al. 2015). Of 469 patients intubated by the physician – paramedic enhanced care team, the ambulance service personnel on scene had been unable to successfully manage the airway in 57 % of cases (269 patients), with complete airway obstruction observed in 16 patients, partial airway obstruction in 158 patients, airway contamination in 159 patients, and oesophageal intubation in 7 patients. This supports the need for enhanced care teams with ability to provide advanced airway interventions, and demonstrates that the airway management requirements of a significant proportion of severely injured trauma patients are not met by current ambulance service interventions.

1.3.4   Who Should Perform PHA?

PHA is not a single-person intervention; therefore this question refers to who should be in the PHA team. The restrictions on UK paramedic practice means that one member of the team must be a physician if PHA is to be undertaken. Therefore, UK HEMS/enhanced care teams are comprised of a physician working in partnership with an experienced paramedic, who has undergone additional advanced skills training for the role. This is similar in Australia and has become accepted practice since an early paper reported an increased rate of intervention when a physician was included in the helicopter rescue team (51 % vs. 10 % intubation, 12 % vs. 1 % thoracostomy) and delivered a significantly reduced mortality (Garner et al. 1999).

Contrary to many countries, HEMS in Germany is exclusively physician-staffed. A paper by Andruszkow et al. (2013) reviewed 13,200 patients with traumatic injuries who were transported by either land paramedics or HEMS. They concluded that although HEMS patients were more seriously injured and had a significantly higher incidence of multiple organ dysfunction and sepsis, these patients demonstrated a survival benefit.

A more recent retrospective observational study from The Netherlands, calculated an additional 5.33 lives saved per 100 dispatches of a physician-staffed HEMS vs. Paramedic emergency medical service (EMS) care (Den Hartog et al. 2015). In this service the HEMS team consists of a trauma surgeon or anaesthetist, working with a specialist nurse and pilot, to bring advanced specialised medical care to the scene, which among other interventions includes advanced airway management, surgical airway and PHA, otherwise not available from the EMS crews.

So, we believe that the PHA team should include a physician; but what specialty should they be trained in? PHA is one of the most complex and involved procedures that can be performed in the pre-hospital environment (Box 1.2).

Box 1.2: Skills Required for PHA
- Technical skills to complete over 100 specific steps
- Cognitive skills to assess patient status and the appropriateness of the intervention
- Judgment to decide the appropriate time to initiate the procedure
- Problem-solving skills to manage critical incidents and patient deterioration

---

PHA requires a degree of self-confidence and this will be enhanced by training and experience. This must be tempered by a respect for the risks involved and the potential for worsening patient outcome. Given the potential for difficult intubating conditions, discussed previously, and the in-hospital studies, which show that anaesthetists generally achieve better laryngoscopic views and more first time intubations, it may appear that PHA should ideally be performed by an anaesthetist. However, some of the in-hospital studies discussed earlier showed that senior EM physicians can perform RSI in the ED with similar success to anaesthetists. In addition, there are several other parts to medical care in the pre-hospital environment, which would not be within the competence or experience of many anaesthetists.

Currently most physicians working within UK HEMS and pre-hospital enhanced care teams are from either EM with additional anaesthesia training or anaesthesia with additional

EM training. Other physicians involved include general practitioners (GPs) and a smaller number of surgeons, who have
undertaken additional training to ensure a comparable skill
set. All physicians must also undertake training and gain
experience of working in the pre-hospital environment.

A number of organisations have published their pre-
hospital intubation practices including the success rates of
physicians from different base specialties. They include the
rates of intubation success, and the frequency and management of failed intubation, as a quality marker of the care
delivered.

The largest of these was the observational study by
London HEMS, documenting 7252 patients requiring
advanced airway management between 1991 and 2012
(Lockey et al. 2014). An immediate surgical airway was performed in 46 (0.6 %) patients, tracheal intubation was successful in 7158 patients (99.3 % of intubation attempts), and
rescue techniques were successfully performed in the other
52 patients. Anaesthetists attempted intubation in 2587
patients and failed in 11 (0.4 %) whilst non-anaesthetists
attempted 4394 intubations and failed in 41 (0.9 %) cases
(P = 0.02). A subset of the same database (2006–2007) analysed the effect of base specialty and stage of training (Harris
and Lockey 2011). All groups achieved a high rate of
intubation success in the first two attempts (98.3–100 %),
although anaesthetic registrars, anaesthetic consultants and
EM consultants all achieved significantly more intubations
on first attempt than EM registrars. It was also shown that
spending less than 6 months in an anaesthetic/intensive care
training post was associated with a significantly lower first
pass intubation rate, in comparison with those who had spent
more than 6 months in such posts.

Breckwoldt et al. (2012) considered physicians working on
the mobile intensive care unit and HEMS from one hospital
in Berlin, to be either 'proficient performers' or 'experts' in
tracheal intubation, based on the Dreyfus and Dreyfus
framework of expertise (novice, competence, proficiency,
expertise and mastery). All physicians had at least 5 years

clinical experience before working pre-hospital. The 'proficient' group were non-anaesthetists and had an average experience of 18 intubations per year, whilst the 'expert' group were anaesthetists and had average experience of 304 intubations per year. 'Experts' were found to have a significantly lower incidence of difficult endotracheal intubation, and a lower (although non-significant) incidence of unexpected difficult intubation.

A 5-year (2003–2009) retrospective review of RSIs performed by the physician-paramedic team of the Warwickshire and Northamptonshire Air Ambulance, demonstrated a 97 % success rate for intubation within two laryngoscopy attempts (194 of 200 RSIs) (Fullerton et al. 2011). Of the six failed intubations, three required >2 laryngoscopy attempts, one utilised an LMA, and two a rescue surgical airway. In comparison to anaesthetists, non-anaesthetists were seen to have a higher (although non-significant) rate of failed intubation.

Chesters et al. (2014) reported 88 RSIs undertaken by the East Anglian Air Ambulance during 2010–2012, with no failed intubations. They found a similar incidence of grade 1 views on laryngoscopy between anaesthetic and EM registrars (40.5 vs. 48.4 %), and between anaesthetic and EM consultants (70 vs. 77.8 %).

The West Midlands Medical Emergency Response Incident Team (MERIT), in their first year of operation (2012–2013), reported 142 RSIs with one case of failure to intubate requiring insertion of a supraglottic airway device (McQueen et al. 2015). Interestingly within this scheme, which operates with a physician – paramedic team, over a third of patients were intubated by the critical care paramedic. All operators displayed similar level of proficiency at obtaining a grade 1 or 2 view on laryngoscopy, regardless of physician base specialty or profession, with the one failed intubation involving an EM registrar. Information regarding the anticipated difficulty of intubation and choice of operator for laryngoscopy is not stated, and therefore it is not known if cases involving anticipated difficulties were deferred to the physician. They conclude that 'the system employed by pre-hospital teams rather than the background of the operator underpins success and proficiency in pre-hospital RSI'.

It is reassuring for clinicians practising PHA, that despite the challenges of performing the procedure in the pre-hospital environment, intubation success rates are high, regardless of background specialty, and comparable to those within hospital practice. Whilst many studies do not demonstrate statistically significant differences between base specialties, it is suggested that anaesthetists tend to gain a better view on laryngoscopy, and have a higher rate of initial attempt success. As may be expected, there appears to be a level of experience that correlates with increased success. For non-anaesthetic physicians, this includes a period of at least 6 months training in anaesthetics, and opportunities to maintain these skills.

In 2009, the Pre-hospital Anaesthesia working party from the Association of Anaesthetists of Great Britain and Ireland (AAGBI) produced guidelines for the conduct of PHA (AAGBI 2009). These outline standards for training, equipment, monitoring, drugs, transport, organisational governance, as well as guidance on techniques and paediatric PHA.

The guidelines state that PHA 'should be performed only by appropriately trained and competent practitioners working in a properly structured pre-hospital system'. The precise level of training and competence is not defined, but it is stated that ability to perform safe PHA should be defined by skills in anaesthesia and working in the pre-hospital environment, rather than the primary specialty of the individual. The Acute Care Common Stem (ACCS) programme which includes 6 months each of EM and acute medicine and 1 year in anaesthesia and intensive care medicine (or equivalent training), combined with specific training for working in the pre-hospital environment, is regarded as the absolute minimum required by a physician to practice PHA. Closely supervised working, and assessment of competence in PHA by practising senior clinicians is considered essential. Whether physicians who do not fulfil these criteria, but who already provide pre-hospital anaesthesia, should continue to do so, is down to the experience and judgment of the individual concerned. This should be in agreement with those responsible for pre-hospital clinical governance in the local area.

Recognition of the requirement for physicians to be specifically trained to deliver emergency care in the pre-hospital environment led to the evolution of Pre-Hospital Emergency Medicine (PHEM) as a medical sub-specialty, led by the Intercollegiate Board for Training in Pre-Hospital Emergency Medicine (IBTPHEM). PHEM was approved by the UK General Medical Council as a sub-specialty of EM and Anaesthesia in July 2011, and as a sub-specialty of Intensive Care Medicine and Acute Internal Medicine in October 2013. The PHEM programme offers structured training, with a comprehensive curriculum, covering all aspects of medical care required by seriously ill or injured patients before they reach hospital and during emergency transfer between hospitals (IBTPHEM, 2012). It is entered after 5 years of post-registration training, with the equivalent of ACCS training a requirement to entry. It aims to create practitioners to meet the requirement for enhanced pre-hospital care, as well as improve quality and standards, governance and equity of existing pre-hospital enhanced care.

The importance of training and experience does not apply solely to the physician undertaking PHA. As per standard UK hospital practice, anaesthesia in the pre-hospital environment should occur only in the presence of an appropriately trained assistant. This role is generally taken by a paramedic, working in partnership with the physician to form the HEMS/enhanced care team. The combined skills and experience of such a team are invaluable, particularly in more difficult situations.

1.4 Summary

- The pre-hospital environment is one of the most challenging clinical settings in which to work, and PHA is one of the most complex procedures performed in this environment.

- Successful PHA requires a team with an adequate level of training and experience in both performing emergency anaesthesia and working in the pre-hospital environment.
- The team should ideally include a physician who has a *minimum* of 6-months training in each of: anaesthesia, intensive care, acute medicine and emergency medicine.

References

Andruszkow H, Lefering R, Frink M, et al. Survival benefit of helicopter emergency medical services compared to ground emergency medical services in traumatized patients. Crit Care. 2013;17(3):R124.

Arbabi S, Jurkovich GJ, et al. A comparison of pre-hospital and hospital data in trauma patients. J Trauma. 2004;56:1029–32.

Association of Anaesthetists of Great Britain and Ireland. Prehospital anaesthesia. London; 2009.

Benger J, Hopkinson S. Rapid sequence induction of anaesthesia in UK emergency departments: a national census. Emerg Med J. 2011;28:217–20.

Breckwoldt J, Klemstein S, Brunne B, et al. Expertise in prehospital endotracheal intubation by emergency medicine physicians – comparing 'proficient performers' and 'experts'. Resuscitation. 2012;83:434–9.

Bulger EM, et al. The use of neuromuscular blocking agents to facilitate prehospital intubation does not impair outcome after traumatic brain injury. J Trauma. 2005;58:718–23.

Chesters A, Keefe N, Mauger J, Lockey D. Prehospital anaesthesia performed in a rural and suburban air ambulance service staffed by a physician and paramedic: a 16-month review of practice. Emerg Med J. 2014;31:65–8.

College of Emergency Medicine. Curriculum assessment system for core speciality training ACCS CT1-3 and higher speciality training ST4-6. 2010. Available via http://www.rcem.ac.uk/Training-Exams/Curriculum. Accessed 02 Apr 2015

Cook TM, Woodall N, Haper J, Benger J, on behalf of the Fourth National Audit Project. Major complications of airway management in the United Kingdom: report and findings of the Fourth National Audit Project of the Royal College of Anaesthetists and the Difficult Airway Society. London: The Royal College of Anaesthetists; 2011.

Davis DP, Hoyt DB, Ochs M, et al. The effect of paramedic rapid sequence intubation on outcome in patients with severe traumatic brain injury. J Trauma. 2003;54:444–53.

Davis DP, Peay J, Serrano JA, et al. The impact of aeromedical response to patients with moderate to severe traumatic brain injury. Ann Emerg Med. 2005;46:115–22.

Deakin CD, et al. A critical reassessment of ambulance service airway management in prehospital care: Joint Royal Colleges Ambulance Liaison Committee Airway Working Group, June 2008. Emerg Med J. 2008;27:226–33.

Den Hartog D, Romeo J, Ringburg AN et al (2015) Survival benefit of physician-staffed Helicopter Emergency Medical Services (HEMS) assistance for severely injured patients. Injury. 2015 Jul; 46:1281–6.

Eckstein M, Chan L, Schneir A, Palmer R. Effect of pre-hospital advanced trauma life support on outcomes of major trauma patients. J Trauma. 2000;48:643–8.

Faculty of Intensive Care Medicine. Curriculum and assessment. 2014. Available via http://www.ficm.ac.uk/curriculum-and-assessment. Accessed 2 Apr 2015.

Fullerton JN, Roberts KJ, Wyse M. Should non-anaesthetists perform pre-hospital rapid sequence induction? An observational study. Emerg Med J. 2011;28:428–31.

Garner A, Rashford S, Lee A, Bartolacci R. Addition of physicians to paramedic helicopter services decreases blunt trauma mortality. Aust N Z J Surg. 1999;69:697–701.

Garner AA, Mann KP, Fearnside M, et al. (2015) The head injury retrieval trial (HIRT): A single-centre randomised controlled trial of physician prehospital management of severe blunt head injury compared with management by paramedics only. Emerg Med J. 2015. doi:10.1136/emermed-2014-204390

Gausche M, Lewis RJ, Stratton SJ. Effect of out-of-hospital paediatric endotracheal intubation on survival and neurological outcome: a controlled clinical trial. JAMA. 2000;283:783–90.

Graham CA, et al. Rapid sequence intubation in Scottish urban emergency departments. Emerg Med J. 2003;20:3–5.

Harris T, Lockey D. Success in physician prehospital rapid sequence intubation: what is the effect of base speciality and length of anaesthetic training. Emerg Med J. 2011;28:225–9.

Hedges JR, Dronen SC, Feero S, et al. Succinyl-choline-assisted intubations in pre-hospital care. Ann Emerg Med. 1988;17: 469–72.

Intercollegiate Board for Training in Pre-Hospital Emergency Medicine. Sub-speciality training in Pre-Hospital Emergency Medicine: a guide of trainees, trainers, local education providers, employers and deaneries. 2012. Available via http://www.ibtphem.org.uk. Accessed 2 Apr 2015.

Joint Royal Colleges Ambulance Liaison Committee. UK ambulance services clinical practice guidelines. Bridgwater: Class Publishing; 2013.

Kerslake D, et al. Tracheal intubation in an urban emergency department in Scotland: a prospective, observational study of 3738 intubations. Resuscitation. 2015;89:20–4.

Lockey D, Crewdson K, Weaver A, Davies G. Observational study of the success rates of intubation and failed intubation airway rescue techniques in 7256 attempted intubations of trauma patients by pre-hospital physicians. Br J Anaesth. 2014;113(2):220–5.

Lockey DJ, et al. Advanced airway management is necessary in pre-hospital trauma patients. Br J Anaesth. 2015;114(4):657–62.

Lossius HM, Sollid SJM, Rehn M, Lockey DJ. Revisiting the value of pre-hospital tracheal intubation: an all time systematic literature review extracting the Utstein airway core variables. Crit Care. 2011;15:R26.

McQueen C, et al. Prehospital anaesthesia performed by physician/critical care paramedic teams in a major trauma network in the UK: a 12 month review of practice. Emerg Med J. 2015;32:65–9.

Murray JA. Pre-hospital intubation in patients with severe head injury. J Trauma. 2000;49:1065–70.

National Confidential Enquiry into Patient Outcome and Death. Trauma: who cares? London; 2007.

Reid C, Chan L, Tweeddale M. The who, where, and what of rapid sequence intubation: prospective observational study of emergency RSI outside the operating theater. Emerg Med J. 2004; 21:296–301.

Sellick BA. Cricoid pressure to control regurgitation of stomach contents during induction of anaesthesia. Lancet. 1961;2:404–5.

Sise MJ, et al. Early intubation in the management of trauma patients: Indications and outcomes in 1000 consecutive patients. J Trauma. 2009;66(1):32–40.

Stept WJ, Safar P. Rapid induction – intubation for prevention of gastric content aspiration. Anaesth Anal. 1970;49:633–6.

Stevenson AG, et al. Tracheal intubation in the emergency department: the Scottish district hospital perspective. Emerg Med J. 2007;24:394–7.

Stockinger ZT, McSwain NE. Pre-hospital tracheal intubation for trauma does not improve survival over bag-valve-mask ventilation in trauma patients. J Trauma. 2004;56:531–6.

Taryle DA, Chandler JE, Good JT, et al. Emergency room intubations-complications and survival. Chest. 1979;75:541–3.

Thomas CM. Emergency tracheal intubation: complications associated with repeated laryngoscopic attempts. Anaesth Anal. 2004; 99:607–13.

Wang HE, Davis DP, Wayne MA, Delbridge T. Prehospital rapid-sequence intubation-what does the evidence show? Prehosp Emerg Care. 2004;8:366–77.

Winchell RJ, Hoyt DB. Endotracheal intubation in the field improves survival in patients with severe head injury. Arch Surg. 1997;132: 592–7.

Chapter 2
Indications and Decision Making

By the end of this chapter you should:

- Know the indications and contraindications for pre-hospital anaesthesia (PHA)
- Understand the significance of aspiration
- Appreciate the risks and benefits of PHA
- Know the factors to consider before undertaking PHA

The decision to escalate airway management from basic to advanced is not always clear-cut. The primary aim must always be to maintain reliable airway patency and ensure adequate oxygenation and ventilation in order to prevent hypoxia and hypercarbia. The airway is also at risk from aspiration or soiling from upper airway debris if the laryngeal reflexes are incompetent or rendered ineffective by drugs. In these cases, or if clear indications exist, consideration should be given to endotracheal intubation (Boxes 2.1 and 2.2).

T. Lowes et al., *Pre-Hospital Anesthesia Handbook*,
DOI 10.1007/978-3-319-23090-0_2,
© Springer-Verlag London 2016

Box 2.1: Indications for PHA
- **To Maintain reliable airway patency**
- **Ventilatory insufficiency** –
  - SpO_2 <92 % despite O_2 or impending respiratory collapse due to exhaustion.
  - To control $PaCO_2$ when raised ICP is a concern
- **Preventing Aspiration** – Loss of airway reflexes/ Glasgow coma scale (GCS) rapidly falling or <9.
- **Patients requiring repeated sedation for safe management** – they present a danger to themselves or attending staff
- **Humanitarian reasons** – Severe injuries/pain unlikely to be relieved without excessive doses of opioid.

Box 2.2: Contraindications to PHA
- **Inexperienced team or inadequate equipment**
- **Known anaphylaxis** to one of the drugs required for intubation (although there may be an alternative).
- **Patient anatomy or airway swelling/distortion** – making successful intubation unlikely (Rapid transfer to hospital is preferred; cricothyroidotomy under local anaesthesia may be the safest technique if respiratory failure develops)
- **Croup or epiglottitis** – failed intubation attempts may leave a critical situation – adrenaline (epinephrine) nebulisers and rapid transfer to hospital preferred.

2.1   Significance of Aspiration

Many patients with a reduced GCS are intubated to 'protect their airway'. The aim is to remove the potential for aspiration in someone who has lost their airway reflexes. The significance of aspiration in the pre-hospital environment is unclear. The risk of aspiration is dependent on both the absence of effective airway reflexes and the presence of something to aspirate (e.g. blood or gastric contents). Death due to aspiration usually occurs in two ways: Large aspirates may cause upper or lower airway obstruction and asphyxiation. Smaller volumes may lead to early hypoxia with subsequent brain death or multiorgan failure. Small aspirates may also cause pneumonia or pneumonitis, with death secondary to sepsis or acute respiratory distress syndrome (ARDS).

2.1.1 Incidence, Morbidity and Mortality of Aspiration

The incidence of aspiration in non-survivors from trauma has been reported to be up to 55 % (where aspiration was defined as the presence of blood, vomit or other material in the upper respiratory tract at post-mortem) (Yates 1977). Ottosson (1985) noted that 20 % of road traffic fatalities had evidence of aspiration, however, it was suggested that the aspiration did not alter the final outcome, as all victims except one had virtually unsurvivable injuries. McNicholl (1994) looked at 239 patients who sustained major trauma (injury severity score >15) and reached hospital alive. Fifteen patients (6 %) aspirated; all before ambulance arrival, and all subsequently died. All of these patients had either severe brain injury or were considered unsalvageable.

So, although Yates' study could suggest that aspiration may be a major contributor to trauma deaths, other studies suggest it is simply a marker of injury severity and an indicator of poor outcome (i.e. more severely injured patients, who are more likely to die, are more prone to aspiration).

In one study of intubation, the incidence of aspiration in those intubated on scene was shown to be significantly greater (50 % vs. 22 %) compared with those intubated in the Emergency department (ED) (Ufberg et al. 2005). As paramedics tend to only intubate those with very low GCS pre-hospital, this may simply confirm that those who are most severely injured are likely to have aspirated by the time a pre-hospital team arrives. This appears to be supported by Lockey et al (2013), who presented a series of 400 patients intubated by a physician led pre-hospital trauma team in London. They found that 177 patients (44 %) had gross airway contamination at the time of intubation. Patients with GCS 3–8 were significantly more likely to have a contaminated airway (57 %) compared with patients of GCS 9–15 (34 %). The contamination was predominantly from upper airway blood (78 %) rather than gastric content and much of this may have appeared in the oropharynx during induction, secondary to ongoing bleeding in facial injuries. Vadeboncoeur et al (2006) noted that aspiration had occurred in 72/269 (27 %) of head-injured patients with GCS <9, prior to intubation. There was only one reported case of aspiration *during* intubation.

It should now be appreciated that strong pre-hospital evidence to recommend intubation as a means to prevent aspiration and reduce mortality does not exist and that aspiration is likely to have already occurred in the majority of those at risk.

There will be a number of patients, however, whose GCS may be deteriorating (combined with a reduction in protective airway reflexes) and who may become at risk of aspiration during transfer due to the presence of blood from facial trauma or regurgitation of gastric contents. In these patients the following statistics should be considered: Perioperative aspiration is associated with around 4 % mortality (Kluger and Short 1999; Warmer et al. 1993), and patients who aspirate have a longer Intensive Care Unit stay and poorer neurological outcome (Bronchard et al. 2004) when compared with those that do not, despite comparable injuries.

Given this information, it would seem reasonable to try and prevent aspiration where possible.

2.2   Laryngeal Mask Airway (LMA) vs. Endotracheal Tube (ETT)

In patients who have evidence of airway soiling, the majority of debris originates from the mouth or nose, with a low incidence of soiling from gastric contents (McNicholl 1994;

Lockey et al. 1999, 2013). This suggests that a laryngeal mask airway (LMA), which provides some protection from soiling from above, may provide reasonable protection in the majority. It will certainly provide more airway protection than when ventilating with only a bag-valve-mask (BVM). It should be remembered, however, that the act of inserting an LMA without prior administration of drugs may provoke vomiting or regurgitation. As a rule, if the level of consciousness has allowed the placement of an oropharyngeal airway, an LMA will usually be tolerated.

2.2.1   Pharmacologically Assisted LMA Insertion (PALM)

A consensus meeting of the Faculty of Pre-Hospital Care was held in April 2012 to discuss the merits of pharmacologically assisted LMA insertion (PALM). The Faculty subsequently published a consensus statement supported by all participating organisations, other than the Royal College of Anaesthetists (Moss et al 2013). PALM was defined as the use of intravenous sedation, without neuromuscular blockade, to facilitate the insertion of a supraglottic airway device (SAD).

Published evidence for the safe pre-hospital use of PALM is limited to a single case series of five patients, and one of these was not actually pharmacologically assisted (Mason 2009). The device used was a single-use intubating-LMA (LMA Fastrach™). In each case the patient was sitting trapped in a vehicle with a reduced SpO_2 despite additional oxygen provided via a face mask or BVM. Three patients had a GCS of 3 with lung contusions, and the other two patients had facial injuries requiring frequent suctioning of blood from the airway. Intravenous Midazolam was used for sedation in four patients and LMA placement was successful in all. Ketamine has been mentioned as an alternative sedative; it may have beneficial cardiovascular effects, however, it may also increase the incidence of laryngospasm and airway secretions.

An earlier paper from Germany reported the successful use of the LMA Fastrach™ by pre-hospital emergency physicians who were encouraged to use it as the first alternative in case of difficult or failed laryngoscopy (Timmerman et al. 2007). Insertion was successful in all 11 patients where the LMA was used (of 146 requiring advanced airway management).

The consensus statement applied strict criteria to the use of PALM, specifying that the use of the technique within a region must be agreed by the local ambulance service medical director (Moss et al 2013). The individual clinician must also be competent in the insertion of the SAD by either routine use as part of their clinical practice or through experience in a supervised clinical setting. Furthermore, the clinician must be competent in; managing ongoing sedation, transfer of a critically ill patient and managing adverse events. The consensus statement made it clear that PALM is a rescue technique to be used only in rare circumstances in a patient with a severely compromised airway where all other simple airway manoeuvres and adjuncts have been exhausted and pre-hospital rapid sequence intubation is not an option.

There are two main concerns with the technique as described. Firstly, intravenous sedation in the sitting position is likely to cause a reduction in blood pressure due to vasodilation and a reduction in venous return. The addition of positive pressure ventilation will further exacerbate this. The subsequent reduction in cerebral perfusion pressure may then negate any benefit from improved oxygen saturation. Secondly, the intravenous sedation is very likely to depress respiratory effort; if the insertion of the LMA is not successful there will be a rapid deterioration in oxygen saturation and potentially an urgent requirement for a surgical airway.

An alternative technique that avoids both issues and may be preferred in a sitting spontaneously breathing patient with airway compromise, is a planned surgical airway. This can be done using local anaesthetic, along with titrated Ketamine to manage agitation. It avoids any depression of respiratory effort and reduction in blood pressure. The preferred technique where possible is, however, prompt extrication followed by rapid sequence intubation (RSI).

2.3 Summary

The question remains whether the risks of an unprotected airway and potential aspiration (or further aspiration) justify the unproven benefit of intubating a patient prior to admission to hospital. As most airway soiling is caused by blood, a simple airway with adequate suction may be sufficient. Adequate oxygenation and ventilation may, however, require an endotracheal tube. An endotracheal tube is the gold standard for airway protection, but strong benefit pre-hospital has yet to be shown.

2.4 Assessment of Need: Risk vs. Benefit

When making an assessment of the requirement for intubation it is important to balance the benefits of the intervention against the risks of performing it (Boxes 2.3 and 2.4).

Box 2.3: Benefits of Intubation
- Provides a secure airway
- Allows ventilation with no leak and also avoids gastric distension
- Allows administration of high FiO_2 and positive end-expiratory pressure (PEEP)
- Provides protection to lungs from soiling with gastric contents and blood
- Allows bronchial suctioning

Box 2.4: Risks of Intubation
- May lead to loss of airway and cerebral injury or death.
- May be complicated by periods of hypoxia or hypercapnia.
- Oesophageal intubation, if unrecognised, will be fatal.
- Endobronchial intubation may result in deterioration rather than improvement in oxygenation.
- Trauma to the airway including teeth, pharynx, larynx, and trachea.
- Worsening of airway obstruction if intubation fails (e.g. burns, epiglottitis).
- Coughing and gagging leading to an increase in intra cranial pressure (ICP).
- Regurgitation or vomiting during the procedure increasing the risk of airway soiling.
- Cardio-vascular instability resulting from laryngoscopy or drug administration.
- Barotrauma due to the application of high airway pressures during ventilation resulting in pneumothorax or tensioning of a simple pneumothorax.

2.4.1   Factors to Consider (The A B C D Approach)

2.4.1.1   Airway

It can be difficult to assess if the airway reflexes are intact. The gag reflex may be absent in 37 % of otherwise healthy people (Davies et al. 1995). Attempting to elicit the reflex may stimulate vomiting and is not recommended. Absence of pharyngeal sensation is a more specific test for risk of aspiration. The presence of swallowing and the ability to clear secretions from the upper airway is therefore a more useful sign and implies coordinated upper airway function. Conscious patients with oral blood from maxillo-facial trauma may be managed best by sitting them forward and escorting them to hospital (with cervical protection if indicated).

2.4.1.2   Breathing

Hypoxia may result from chest pathology or inadequate ventilation. A physical examination may reveal treatable causes and these should be immediately addressed (e.g., tension pneumothorax). The patient with a large open pneumothorax may entrain air through their wound rather than down their trachea whilst spontaneously breathing. These patients should be managed by applying a self-adhesive one-way valve (e.g. Bolin/ Russell chest seal), or occlusive dressing and chest drain. Intubation may then not be required. Improvements in oxygenation and ventilation can be achieved from the provision of analgesia or by altering the patients' position (uninjured side uppermost). Sitting the patient up can also improve respiratory dynamics and can be useful for left ventricular failure.

2.4.1.3   Circulation

Intravenous access was previously a prerequisite for PHA, but adult intraosseous access devices are now available and can offer a reliable alternative to cannulation. Suitable sites include the sternum, humerus and tibia, and PHA can safely be performed using this approach.

Hypovolaemic patients will become hypotensive after induction. A reduced dose of induction agent should be considered (see Chap. 7). Fluid bolus and/or vasopressors should be prepared and given as required. Immediate transfer to definitive care for early surgery without intubation may be indicated. This is particularly applicable to patients with blunt abdominal trauma and non-compressible haemorrhage. These patients can decompensate markedly after induction. This can result from a combination of: reduced endogenous catecholamines, drug-induced vasodilation and myocardial depression, the loss of abdominal muscle tone (tamponade effect) and reduced venous return following positive pressure ventilation. Severe hypotension and cardiac arrest can swiftly follow. Delaying PHA until the patient is in the operating theatre with a surgeon ready to perform a laparotomy may be the best option.

2.4.1.4   Disability

A GCS of less than 9, or a progressive deterioration in the score, is a strong indication for intubation. Agitation or aggression may necessitate the need for sedation and intubation to safely transport a patient. It should be remembered, however, that intubation to make an otherwise stable patient suitable for air transfer may be inappropriate if a ground vehicle is available and an appropriate receiving hospital is within a short travelling time.

In addition to assessing A, B, C, and D, the following points need consideration:

- The environment and its suitability for the intervention
- The team's expertise and available personnel (minimum of one assistant required)
- The distance to definitive care and the speed and means of transfer
- The availability of equipment (minimum monitoring standards are required)
- The significance of not intervening

2.5   Summary

- The priority in pre-hospital care is to ensure a patent airway and adequate ventilation.
- The risk and benefit should be considered prior to intubation for each patient.

References

Bronchard R, Albaladejo P, Brezac G, Geffroy A, Seine PF. Early onset pneumonia: risk factors and consequences in head trauma patients. Anaesthesiology. 2004;100:234–9.

Davies AE, Kidd D, Stone SP, MacMahon J. Pharyngeal sensation and gag reflex in healthy subjects. Lancet. 1995;345:487–8.

Kluger MT, Short TG. Aspiration during anaesthesia: a review of 133 cases from the Australian Anaesthetic Incident Monitoring study (AIMS). Anaesthesia. 1999;54:19–26.

Lockey DJ, Coats T, Parr MJA. Aspiration in severe trauma: a prospective study. Anaesthesia. 1999;54:1097–8.

Lockey DJ, Avery P, Harris T, Davies GE, Lossius HM. A prospective study of physician pre-hospital anaesthesia in trauma patients: oesophageal intubation, gross airway contamination and the 'quick look' airway assessment. BMC Anesthesiol. 2013;13:21.

Mason AM. Prehospital use of the intubating laryngeal mask airway in patients with severe polytrauma: a case series. Case Rep Med. 2009. doi:10.1155/2009/938531.

McNicholl BP. The golden hour and pre-hospital care. Injury. 1994;25:251–4.

Moss R, Porter K, Greaves I. Pharmacologically assisted laryngeal mask insertion: a consensus statement. Emerg Med J. 2013;30:1073–5.

Ottosson A. Aspiration and obstructed airways as the cause of death in 158 consecutive traffic fatalities. J Trauma. 1985;25:538–40.

Timmerman A, Russo SG, Rosenblatt WH, et al. Intubating laryngeal mask airway for difficult out-of-hospital airway management: a prospective evaluation. Br J Anaesth. 2007;99:286–91.

Ufberg JW, Bushra JS, Karras DJ, Satz WA, Kueppers F. Aspiration of gastric contents: association with prehospital intubation. Am J Emerg Med. 2005;23:379–82.

Vadeboncoeur TF, et al. The ability of paramedics to predict aspiration in patients undergoing prehospital rapid sequence intubation. J Emerg Med. 2006;30:131–6.

Warmer MA, Warmer ME, Weber JG. Clinical significance of pulmonary aspiration during the perioperative period. Anaesthesiology. 1993;78:56–62.

Yates DW. Airway patency in fatal accidents. Br Med J. 1977;2:1249–51.

Chapter 3
Pre-hospital Rapid Sequence Intubation (PRSI)

By the end of this chapter you will be able to:

- List the six P's of PRSI
- Discuss each of the P's in turn
- Appreciate the importance of a plan D

3.1   The Six P's (Fig. 3.1)

PRSI can be separated into six phases:

1. Preoxygenation
2. Preparation
3. Premedication
4. Paralysis and Sedation
5. Passage of the Endotracheal tube
6. Post intubation care

It is important that each member of the team is familiar with all phases of PRSI. This allows preparation to take place concurrently with ongoing patient management.

T. Lowes et al., *Pre-Hospital Anesthesia Handbook*,
DOI 10.1007/978-3-319-23090-0_3,
© Springer-Verlag London 2016

Preoxygenation	High flow O_2 with reservoir mask or BVM
Preparation	Preassessment <C> ABCDE Prepare equipment and drugs (PRSI checklist) Position patient and team Protect (c-spine & cricoid pressure)
Premedication	Fentanyl 0–3 mcg/kg
Paralyse & sedate	Induction drug Neuromuscular blocking agent Cricoid pressure
Pass the ETT	Use a bougie Locate vocal cords and place ETT Consider BURP or ease cricoid pressure Failed Intubation procedures
Post intubation care	Inflate cuff, Confirm placement (Cricoid pressure off), Secure ETT Check observations Continue sedation and paralysis ABCDEF pre-transfer checks Transfer to hospital

FIGURE 3.1   The 6 P's

3.2   Preoxygenation

This is an essential phase in the conduct of safe PRSI. It provides an oxygen safety buffer to prevent precipitous desaturation occurring in the period of hypoventilation and apnoea, prior to and during laryngoscopy. Desaturation below an oxygen saturation (SpO_2) of 70 %, places patients at risk of cardiovascular instability, hypoxic organ damage and death (Mort 2004).

Desaturation is a significant complication of PRSI. The Scottish Emergency Medical Retrieval Service found that 15.4 % (32 of 208 patients) had a desaturation episode during the procedure (below 90 % or a reduction in >10 % from initial SpO_2) (Wimalasena et al. 2014).

The aim of preoxygenation is to replace the air in the alveoli with an enriched oxygen mixture, particularly in the functional residual capacity of the lungs. This will act as a reservoir for the body during apnoea. In ideal conditions this offers several minutes before desaturation occurs (Fig. 3.2, Box 3.1). Unfortunately, conditions for PRSI are rarely ideal, and critically ill patients with increased metabolic demand, hypovolaemia, reduced cardiac output and possible lung injury will desaturate far quicker than this.

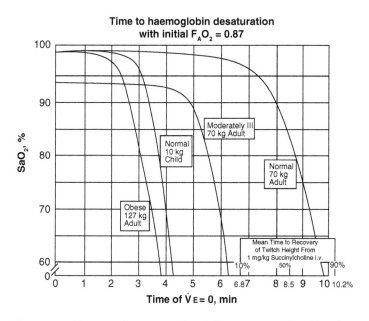

FIGURE 3.2 Desaturation curves after full pre-oxygenation (Fraction Alveolar Oxygen = 0.87) (Benumof et al. 1997)

Box 3.1: Approximate Time for Desaturation to 90 % After Full Preoxygenation (Benumof et al. 1997)
- Normal 70 kg adult = 8 min
- Moderately ill 70 kg adult = 4.8 min
- Normal 10 kg child = 3.4 min
- Obese 127 kg adult = 2.6 min

3.2.1 Preoxygenation Strategies

Preoxygenation should be performed using a tight-fitting face mask with a reservoir and ≥15 L/min of oxygen in order to provide a high (>0.9) fraction of inspired oxygen (FiO_2) during inspiration. In hospital this is done using either a standard anaesthetic circuit or a disposable Mapleson C (sometimes called a 'Waters' circuit) with adjustable pressure limiting (APL) valve (Fig. 3.3). This also allows an element of

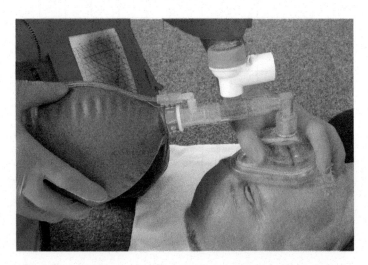

Figure 3.3 Mapleson C circuit With adjustable pressure limiting (APL) valve being used to apply CPAP

continuous positive airway pressure (CPAP) to be applied, as long as the face mask is tight-fitting. These systems require a constant high flow of oxygen and a tight seal to allow manual ventilation, neither of which can be guaranteed in the pre-hospital setting. The default system in the emergency situation is a self-inflating bag-valve-mask (BVM), of which there are many varieties, including many single-use versions. Some older versions of BVMs did not have one-way exhalation valves near the mask and therefore allowed entrainment of air into the face mask at lower oxygen flow rates. These would deliver relatively low FiO_2 (<0.4) during spontaneous ventilation (Mills et al. 1991; Nimmagadda et al. 2000). This is not the case with the majority of BVM systems currently in use, however, it is always important to check the type of BVM being used.

Even when a BVM has a one-way exhalation valve, there is variation in the FiO_2 delivered by different BVM systems in common use. As an example, two single-use BVMs with exactly 15 L/min of oxygen attached, were compared for both ease of breathing and delivered FiO_2 (using a calibrated oxygen analyser in a t-piece behind the face mask).

The Ambu Single Patient Use Resuscitator (SPUR) II (Fig. 3.4a) has an extremely low resistance inspiratory/expiratory single-shutter (one-way) valve at the patient end (Fig. 3.4b) which provided only minimal resistance to breathing. The valve prevents entrainment of air during inhalation, so only oxygen from the bag is inhaled if the mask is correctly sealed on the patient's face. Even during large inspiratory breaths, the FiO_2 remained above 0.9 at all times and at normal tidal volumes was 0.95. The large safety inspiratory valve at the reservoir bag end of the BVM assembly (Fig. 3.4c) is designed to allow air to be entrained if the reservoir bag is completely empty, to prevent asphyxiation. This only opened a little even during large tidal volumes; hence the FiO_2 only dropped slightly due to indrawn air mixing with the oxygen.

The Marshall Classic Manual Resuscitator (Fig. 3.5a) has a Laerdal type 'duck-billed' inspiratory valve and a flat silicone

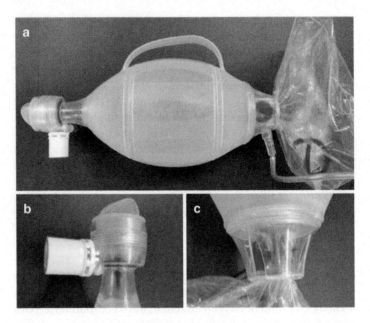

FIGURE 3.4 (a) Ambu SPUR II, (b) Single Shutter inspiratory/expiratory valve. (c) Inspiratory safety valve

ring one-way expiratory valve at the patient end (Fig. 3.5b). The 'duck-billed' valve is subjectively more difficult to breathe through. The additional negative pressure generated, along with the small size and lightweight safety inspiratory valve (Fig. 3.5c), means that air is entrained through the valve even during relatively small volume breaths. This reduced the measured FiO_2 from 0.9 at normal tidal volume down to 0.75 during larger inspiratory breaths. It is useful to know that both the ease of breathing and the inspired FiO_2 can be improved significantly by gently squeezing the bag in time with the patient's inspiration.

Even more important than the design of the valves is a good seal between the mask and the patient's face. Gas will always take the path of least resistance. During inspiration with a poor seal, gas will be entrained around the edges of

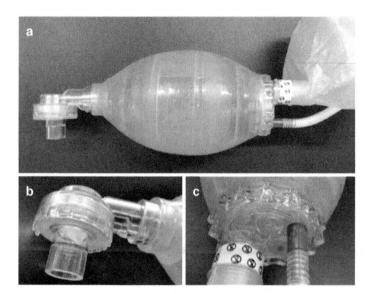

FIGURE 3.5 (**a**) Marshall Classic Resuscitator, (**b**) 'Duck-billed' inspiratory valve. (**c**) Inspiratory safety valve

the mask rather than drawing from the oxygen in the bag and reservoir via the one-way inspiratory valve. The requirement for a good face seal also applies to disposable non-rebreathe reservoir masks; the path of least resistance is also around the edge of the mask rather than through the one-way valve (although the resistance through the valve does tend to be less than in a BVM).

With a good seal and a patient with reasonable inspiratory effort, a BVM with a reservoir bag and >15 L/min will provide a high FiO_2 (>0.9) and avoids the requirement to change face mask during the RSI (Nimmagadda et al. 2000). It also means that ventilation can be easily assisted if inspiratory breaths are shallow or if SpO_2 drops whilst waiting for the muscle relaxant to work.

BVM preoxygenation does, however, require a competent additional person to maintain the tight face seal whilst the team is preparing for RSI. It may be more practical (and also possibly less daunting for the patient), to use a well-fitting 'non-rebreathe' face mask with reservoir bag for preoxygenation. This is held in place with an elastic strap placed behind the head. Basic models are not ideal as they have a thin plastic edge that may not create a good seal, and an open hole in one side of the mask that allows air to be entrained if the oxygen supply fails (Fig. 3.6). Both of these factors can result in a relatively low FiO_2 (0.6–0.7), even at very high oxygen flow rates. Newer rebreathe masks have softer cushioned edges, which improve the seal, and have no open

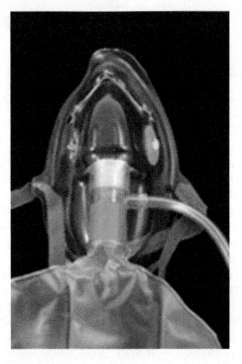

Figure 3.6 Basic non-rebreathe mask

holes in the sides of the mask, thereby increasing the chance of delivering an FiO_2 closer to 0.9 whilst freeing up an extra person (Fig. 3.7). With additional nasal cannula oxygen, as described below, this can increase the FiO_2 further (Fig. 3.8). Clearly if the patient requires assistance to maintain airway patency or needs assisted ventilation, this benefit of freeing a person is lost.

Three minutes of normal tidal volume breaths is acceptable preoxygenation for most patients. This preoxygenation can be improved by asking the patient to fully exhale and

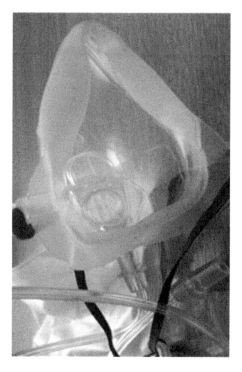

FIGURE 3.7 Newer non-rebreathe mask

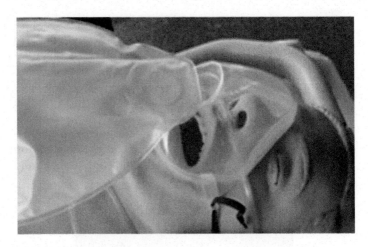

FIGURE 3.8 Non-rebreathe oxygen mask with additional nasal cannula in place for apnoeic oxygenation during PRSI

inhale (vital capacity breaths), although most patients in the pre-hospital setting are unable to co-operate with such a request. Analgesia prior to preoxygenation may improve the effectiveness by reducing pain from chest trauma and increasing inspiratory volumes.

In agitated patients it may be necessary to use sedation to facilitate preoxygenation. Small doses of Midazolam (1–2 mg) or Ketamine (10–40 mg) should be titrated to effect. Weingart et al (2015) reported the successful use of Ketamine 1 mg/kg (+/− further 0.5 mg/kg aliquots) to facilitate preoxygenation in agitated patients. This then allowed 3 min of pre-oxygenation, before full sedation and a muscle relaxant were given. Although based on a relatively small convenience sample of patients unable to tolerate preoxygenation due to delirium, they demonstrated the ability to increase mean pre-laryngoscopy SpO_2 from 89.9 to 98.8 %, and reported no complications such as pre-muscle relaxant apnoea, peri-intubation emesis, cardiac arrest or death, from doing so. Preoxygenation was achieved with a high flow non-rebreathe oxygen mask, or non-invasive CPAP if SpO_2 <95 %. They commented that facilitating preoxygenation in this manner avoids the risks of proceeding to RSI without an adequate oxygen reserve in the patient, and the potential risks of peri-intubation BVM ventilation that may be required to prevent desaturation; such as gastric insufflation and aspiration. They termed this 'delayed sequence intubation' although it is essentially just sedation to facilitate preoxygenation. This concept has been advocated on the PHA course for several years.

SpO_2 will fall precipitously during the 45–60 s of apnoea whilst awaiting onset of muscle relaxation, if starting SpO_2 is already low. In these patients, if already receiving oxygen through a BVM, it may be advisable to gently augment the patient's own respiratory effort prior to induction in order to maintain a safe oxygen saturation throughout the procedure. CPAP can also be applied to improve oxygenation if it is possible to fit an external positive end expiratory pressure (PEEP) valve to the BVM.

If ventilation is continued following induction and apnoea, cricoid pressure will help to avoid the associated gastric insufflation and reduce the risk of aspiration, although this may make ventilation more difficult in some cases. BVM ventilations should aim to be delivered slowly with both low volume (6–7 mL/kg) and low rate, in order to avoid inspiratory pressures sufficient to overcome the lower oesophageal sphincter pressure.

There is evidence that head-up positioning delays the time to desaturation during apnoea (Lane et al. 2005; Ramkumar et al. 2011). It may also reduce the risk of passive regurgitation. This may be achieved by using a semi-recumbent position on a stretcher trolley or, in trauma patients requiring spinal immobilisation, a reverse-trendelenburg position, with the head of the spinal board/scoop stretcher/trolley raised 30° above the feet.

3.2.2   Apnoeic Oxygenation

Although described in the medical literature for over a century, the application of apnoeic oxygenation to pre-hospital airway management procedures is relatively recent (Weingart et al. 2011). It utilises the physiological principle that even without respiratory effort, approximately 250 mL/min oxygen is taken from the alveoli into the bloodstream. If oxygen is supplied to a patent upper airway, a mass flow of gas from the pharynx to alveoli maintains this diffusion of oxygen into the bloodstream, and in doing so, maintains oxygenation without ventilation. The Greater Sydney Helicopter Emergency Medical Service (HEMS) has included apnoeic oxygenation in their PRSI standard operating procedure (SOP) since 2011. During the preoxygenation phase, whilst a non-rebreather mask or BVM set at 15 L/min oxygen is used to preoxygenate, nasal cannulae are applied and set to 5 L/min oxygen, as tolerated (Fig. 3.8). After induction drugs are administered, the flow rate of the nasal cannulae is increased to 15 L/min until the endotracheal tube is secured (Wimalasena et al. 2015). During the 22-month period prior to apnoeic oxygenation, 22.6 % of patients had a desaturation episode below 93 % during RSI, compared to 16.5 % of patients in the 22-month period after introduction of apnoeic oxygenation to the SOP. They suggest this simple and inexpensive technique is of clear clinical benefit to critically ill and injured patients undergoing PRSI.

3.3   Preparation

Performance of a rapid sequence intubation is not immediate and requires time for preparation. The time spent in the preparation phase is never wasted and will increase the chances of a swift and safe intubation. There are four elements to preparation for PRSI (Box 3.2).

Box 3.2: Preparation
- Preassessment
- Prepare equipment and drugs
- Position patient and team
- Protect (c-spine and cricoid pressure)

3.3.1   Preassessment

Preassessment should be easily remembered with a familiar <C>ABCDE approach. It is a similar, but much more rapid assessment, to that which occurs before any anaesthetic in the hospital environment.

3.3.1.1   Catastrophic Haemorrhage

Catastrophic haemorrhage should be controlled at the earliest opportunity during pre-hospital management. This may involve use of wound packing and direct pressure, haemostatic agents and tourniquets. Reducing blood loss and promoting clotting at this earliest stage, not only is beneficial to the patient overall, but also promotes haemodynamic optimisation in preparation for PRSI. Splinting fractures of the pelvis and long bones (particularly femur) is important and will also minimise blood loss, but this occurs after assessment of the Circulation (Sect. 3.3.1.4).

3.3.1.2   Airway

The main concerns are to achieve maximum airway patency to allow preoxygenation prior to RSI, and to be able to predict the likelihood of a "difficult airway."

Difficult Airway

The definition of a difficult airway is that a trained clinician experiences difficulties with mask ventilation, endotracheal intubation or both (American Society of Anesthesiologists (ASA) 2013). Difficult mask ventilation is defined as a situation when it is impossible to maintain SpO_2 above 90 % or it is not possible to reverse signs of inadequate ventilation with a BVM and 100 % oxygen. The incidence of difficulty in airway maintenance in trauma patients can be up to 18 % (Smith and Dejoy 2001). The incidence of a difficult airway is likely to be higher in the pre-hospital environment, for reasons mentioned earlier. Airway assessment should therefore include a judgment of the likely ease of airway maintenance with a BVM, as well as the potential for difficult intubation. The anticipation of difficulty may require a change of the initial management plan (Box 3.3).

Box 3.3: Reasons for Difficulty in Maintaining an Airway
- Obesity
- The presence of a beard
- The edentulous patient
- Facial injury

Difficult Intubation

Difficult intubation is defined in many different ways in various studies, making comparative reporting difficult. The 2013 guidelines of the ASA divide difficult intubation into two parts: difficult laryngoscopy and difficult intubation. Difficult laryngoscopy is defined as being unable to visualise any portion of the vocal cords after multiple attempts at conventional laryngoscopy (i.e. Cormack-Lehane grade ≥ 3 (Fig. 3.20)), and difficult tracheal intubation as the requirement for multiple attempts. (This was previously described by the same group as more than 3 attempts or requiring more than 10 min with conventional laryngoscopy (ASA 1993)). Failed intubation is then described as failure to place the endotracheal tube after multiple attempts (ASA 2013). The widespread use of alternative devices that provide indirect views of the larynx (e.g. Airtraq™ etc.) adds further complexity to these definitions.

The Whatcom Medic One service reported a pre-hospital failed intubation rate of 3.4 % (2978 patients), although some intubated patients required three attempts (Wang et al. 2004). This is identical to the failure rate reported by Fakhry et al. (Fakhry et al. 2006), again a paramedic service allowing up to three attempts at intubation (175 patients). In 1993 London HEMS, a physician led service, reported a requirement for surgical cricothyroidotomy in 7.7 % of 143 patients requiring advanced airway management on scene (Xeropotamos et al. 1993). Since then PRSI training has much improved. The London HEMS data 1991–2012 presented by Lockey et al. (2014) included 7256 patients requiring advanced airway management. An immediate surgical airway was performed in 46 patients (0.6 %), and just 52 of 7210 patients (0.7 %) required a rescue technique for failed intubation.

Breckwoldt et al. (2011) looked to characterise factors contributing to difficult pre-hospital intubation (defined as more than 3 attempts or grade 3 or 4 view) in their physician led teams (2004–2005). In this series of 276 intubation attempts, 3 patients (1.1 %) required a fourth intubation attempt, and 4 patients (1.4 %) required rescue techniques for failed intubation. Difficult intubation (36 patients (13 %)), was significantly associated with short neck, body mass index (BMI) >30, anatomical abnormalities (micrognathia (small lower jaw), ankylosing spondylitis), mouth opening (<3 cm), neck/face trauma, laryngeal oedema, and limited space on scene. Unexpected difficult intubation occurred in 5 % of patients in whom physicians had predicted no difficulties.

In a series of 400 pre-hospital intubations by the physician-led trauma team in London (2007–2008), initial view at laryngoscopy was grade 3 in 12 % of patients and grade 4 in 5 % of patients, although it is not commented upon as to whether an improved view was subsequently achieved (Lockey et al. 2013). Physicians were asked to predict whether laryngoscopy was likely to be difficult, and this

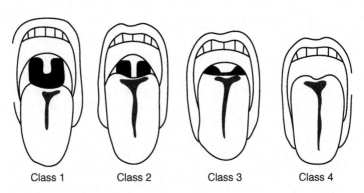

Class 1   Class 2   Class 3   Class 4

FIGURE 3.9 Airway assessment – modified Mallampati classification. The view of the pharyngeal structures is observed, with the mouth open and tongue protruded maximally (Reproduced by kind permission Anaesthesia UK Website)

'quick look' assessment generated sensitivity of 0.597 and specificity of 0.763, with positive predictive value of 0.336 and negative predictive value of 0.904, demonstrating some utility of this method, although not in isolation.

The Modified Mallampati classification of airway assessment (Fig. 3.9) is a commonly used tool in the hospital environment to predict difficult intubation (likelihood of difficulty increases from Class 1 to Class 4). Unfortunately it requires an awake and cooperative patient, so it is usually not useful in patients requiring pre-hospital RSI. Other predictors of difficult intubation may be present (Box 3.4). The 'LEMON' assessment tool, is one system commonly taught for emergency airway assessment which combines most of these factors into a mnemonic (Box 3.5).

Clinical Signs of Potential Difficult Intubation or Ventilation

Obese Patients

Obese patients or those with short muscular necks can be difficult to intubate and ventilate. Excess soft tissue around the airway may hinder displacement during laryngoscopy. This may affect the view. These tissues may also collapse

Box 3.4: Reasons for Difficult Intubation
- Large/prominent upper incisors
- Limited mouth opening
- Reduced range of movement of the head/neck (MILS)
- Reduced sterno-mental distance ("no-neck"), thyro-mental distance ("chinless")
- Swollen/oedematous tongue or laryngeal/pharyngeal tissue
- Congenital abnormalities
- Previous maxillo-facial surgery or radiotherapy

Box 3.5: LEMON Airway Assessment
- **L**ook externally (obesity, short wide neck, small mouth, beard, lower facial trauma, high arched palate, large prominent teeth)
- **E**valuate the 3:3:2 rule (3 cm mouth opening, 3 cm distance tip of chin to hyoid bone, 2 cm between hyoid bone and thyroid notch)
- **M**allampati score
- **O**bstruction (stridor, foreign objects, pooling secretions, neck mass/swelling)
- **N**eck mobility (immobilisation (MILS)/fixation, degenerative disease)

over laryngeal structures making manual ventilation difficult. Two-handed mask ventilation with an oropharyngeal airway may be required.

Edentulous Patients

Edentulous patients are often easy to intubate but can be difficult to manually ventilate. The lack of teeth leaves less support for the cheeks, and as a result the face mask seal may be poor. This can be remedied with a two-handed technique bunching the facial tissue up into the mask to achieve a seal. Again an oropharyngeal airway may make ventilation easier. Early intubation or use of a laryngeal mask airway (LMA) may be required if ventilation is inadequate.

"Chinless" Patients

Patients with micrognathia (receding chin) usually have an anterior larynx. There is a reduced thyromental distance: tip of chin to thyroid cartilage (Adam's apple) of <6.5 cm *with the neck extended*. This measurement is therefore not practical when cervical spine injury is a concern. An impression of micrognathia should still be a visual clue. These patients do not have enough space to displace tissue forward to allow intubation. Laryngeal manipulation such as backward upward rightward pressure (BURP) and a bougie will often be required. (Note: Male patients often grow a beard to hide a small chin).

"No-Neck" Patients

A reduced sternomental distance (tip of chin to sternum <12.5 cm) is predictive of a difficult intubation. Again, this measurement is based on the head in an extended position and is therefore not usually practical. Subjective appearance may add to your assessment of difficulty.

Bearded Patients

As well as sometimes hiding micrognathia, a beard makes it difficult to achieve an adequate seal with a face mask to allow ventilation. Applying lubricating jelly to the beard and using a two-person technique will improve the situation. An LMA may be required to ventilate if intubation is not possible.

"Goofy" Patients

A prominent overbite (protruding upper teeth) can impede laryngoscopy. It may be difficult to manoeuvre the laryngoscope without levering on the upper teeth. External pressure on the larynx (above the cricoid cartilage) i.e. BURP, and use of a Macintosh No. 3 blade, inserted fully inside the mouth (past the top teeth), may help.

"Stiff-Neck" Patients

In patients with poor neck mobility, the larynx will, in effect, be more anterior. In patients with no risk of neck instability, elevating the head further to compensate for reduced extension of the head along with thyroid pressure and a bougie, gives the best chance of success. If there is a chance of underlying instability and risk of spinal cord injury (e.g. severe rheumatoid arthritis), no head or neck movement should take place. The only movement that is appropriate is jaw distraction.

Bleeding (Oral) Patients

Management of patients with blood in the oropharynx can present a particular challenge to the intubator. These patients are best managed in a slightly head-down position. This allows blood to pool in the upper pharynx away from the vocal cords. Adequate suction is the key to success; two suction devices may be required.

Remember A predicted difficult intubation may actually be easy but conversely some "easy" intubations turn out to be difficult. This necessitates the need for a fallback plan or "Plan B" (see text later).

3.3.1.3   Breathing

The initial assessment will have determined the urgency for PRSI. A hypoxic patient with a poor respiratory effort will prompt a more rapid response than one with adequate oxygenation and ventilation but who has a reduced GCS.

If a pneumothorax has been diagnosed, this should have been treated at least with needle thoracocentesis (Appendix

"Needle Thoracocentesis") prior to intubation. Positive pressure ventilation can rapidly change a pneumothorax into a tension pneumothorax, resulting in profound cardiovascular collapse. A thoracostomy ± drain (Appendix "Thoracostomy & Chest Drain Insertion") must be performed immediately after PRSI.

(Note: Thoracostomy without a drain is only permissible in a *ventilated* patient. If the patient is breathing spontaneously, a thoracostomy will create an open pneumothorax, which will not improve ventilation. A valve system to prevent air entrainment during inspiration is therefore required i.e., a chest drain. (A needle/cannula thoracostomy is acceptable before RSI as this allows the release of a "tension" but is too small to allow any significant entrainment of air during inspiration)).

3.3.1.4   Circulation

Intravenous (IV) access is required and should be checked with a 10 mL flush to ensure patency. This must be adequately secured (IV sites are particularly vulnerable in the pre-hospital environment.) Ideally two sites of IV access are obtained prior to RSI in major trauma. This allows rapid infusion of blood products/fluids in one whilst leaving another available for drugs, including those for PHA. It is, however, not always practical or possible due to limb injuries or patient agitation.

In the critically ill patient intraosseous (IO) access may be appropriate if two attempts at IV access have failed or venous access is clearly very poor. Although originally only used in children, adult IO access for emergency resuscitation has become an accepted technique over the last few years, partly due to successes reported in military use (Cooper et al. 2007). IV access is still preferable, as fluids will flow more easily, whereas IO access requires pressurisation of fluid bags or use of a 50 ml syringe and 3-way tap to achieve adequate flow rates for fluid resuscitation. All RSI drugs can be administered via IO access, with intubation success rates (first pass intubation and grade of view) that match those of IV induction (Barnard et al. 2014).

Even in the pre-hospital environment, IV or IO access should be gained as aseptically as possible. Wipes (2 % chlorhexidine in 70 % alcohol) should be used to clean the skin, and minimal handling of the puncture site is advocated. Where asepsis is not possible, it is worth noting this during handover, so the receiving hospital staff can replace it as soon as practical.

Induction of anaesthesia is challenging in the haemodynamically unstable patient, requiring appropriate timing within the resuscitation, and careful drug dosing. The assessment of shock (inadequate tissue perfusion) in the pre-hospital patient can be difficult. Skin colour and capillary return may be misleading in a cold environment. Confusion and level of consciousness may be lost as a guide to adequate perfusion if there is a coexisting head injury. Heart rate can be very useful, but is not specific to changes in volume status. Tachycardia may result from sympathetic stimulation secondary to inadequate analgesia (or sedation when the patient is intubated). Bradycardia may be due to beta-blockers, high spinal cord injury or be may be heralding a pre-terminal event.

In the absence of a measured blood pressure, the presence, site and character of peripheral pulses may give useful information about cardiovascular status (e.g. no palpable radial pulse or a weak/'thready' pulse. It is somotimes said that the presence of a radial pulse implies a blood pressure of 80–90 mmHg and the presence of a carotid pulse equates to a blood pressure of 60–70 mmHg, however, this has not been validated (Greaves et al. 2000). There is no doubt that the presence of a radial pulse implies a higher blood pressure than the presence of a carotid pulse alone.

In the majority of pre-hospital cases, hypotension will be secondary to hypovolaemia. If haemorrhage is external, compressible and controlled, it may be reasonable to give further fluid to aim towards a more normal Mean Arterial Pressure (MAP) for that patient. Conversely, if the hypovolaemia is due to internal, non-compressible haemorrhage, current opinion is that further fluid should be withheld unless the radial pulse becomes impalpable once more (or the blood pressure drops below 80 mmHg systolic/conscious level drops). The reasoning behind this is that an increase in blood pressure may dislodge a newly formed clot, thus resulting in greater loss of blood. In addition, if fluid resuscitation is not with blood products, dilutional coagulopathy will occur. Some UK HEMS units now carry blood products (red cells +/− plasma), and in the bleeding patient this would be used in preference to crystalloid in order to provide more 'haemostatic' resuscitation. In the absence of blood products, a 250 mL bolus of either a 'balanced' crystalloid (e.g. Hartmann's) or 0.9 % NaCl is recommended. Crystalloids are preferred to colloids. A Cochrane Review in 2013 concluded: 'There is no evidence from randomised controlled trials that resuscitation with colloids reduces the risk of death, compared to resuscitation with crystalloids, in patients with trauma, burns or following surgery. Furthermore, the use of hydroxyethyl starch might increase mortality. As colloids are not associated with an improvement in survival and are considerably more expensive than crystalloids, it is hard to see how their continued use in clinical practice can be justified' (Perel et al. 2013).

The concept of allowing the blood pressure to remain low in order to minimise further blood loss is termed 'permissive hypotension'. Prolonged hypotension will, however, increase the likelihood of both multi-organ failure due to hypoperfusion and worsening of coagulopathy due to the 'Acute Coagulopathy of Trauma' (ACoT) (Brohi et al. 2007). ACoT appears to be due to tissue hypoperfusion. This would seem to support previous practice of giving aggressive fluid resuscitation to normalise the blood pressure of a trauma patient, as this should theoretically reduce ACoT. This leaves the pre-hospital practitioner with two apparently conflicting courses of action. The British Military currently advocates 'novel hybrid resuscitation', whereby hypotensive resuscitation is practised for the first hour after injury, followed by normotensive resuscitation. The rationale for this compromise is that clot will form and become sufficiently robust in that first hour, then by increasing blood pressure to allow normal perfusion, ACoT and organ failure should be minimised.

In patients who have sustained a severe head injury, hypotensive resuscitation is not appropriate. These patients may have reduced Cerebral Perfusion Pressure (CPP) secondary to a raised intra cranial pressure (ICP) and a further lowering of MAP would risk cerebral ischaemia. A compromise for patients with severe head injury (GCS <8) *and* ongoing/noncompressible haemorrhage, is a target MAP of >80 mmHg (Spahn et al. 2013).

Hypothermia (<35 °C) will also have an effect on coagulopathy. Ideally all fluids should be warmed and efforts made to minimise heat loss (e.g. reflective/insulated/heat-generating blankets, heated transfer vehicle).

3.3.1.5 Disability

In head-injured patients, particular attention should be placed on pre-sedation pupil responses and GCS, particularly the motor score, as these have the most prognostic significance (along with age and CT scan appearance) (Murray et al. 2007). It should be documented and communicated on hand over.

Level of consciousness may also affect the amount of induction agent given, however it should be remembered that one of the reasons for giving the induction agent is to obtund the hypertensive response to laryngoscopy. This dose may be similar whether the patient is unconscious or not.

3.3.1.6 Exposure

Exposure of the patient may have occurred to varying extents to allow a primary survey to be conducted. Maintaining normothermia of the patient is the target, and it is important to keep the patient protected from the elements where possible. The head and neck will clearly need to be exposed for intubation, as will the chest when confirming position afterwards.

Visualising the larynx is likely to be more difficult in the presence of driving rain, sleet or snow, and unfortunately also in bright direct sunlight. It may be appropriate to move the casualty prior to attempting intubation in adverse weather conditions (e.g. undercover or into an ambulance). Alternatively a ground sheet or similar may be held above the casualty if other emergency service personnel are able to assist. (Note: In certain situations, access to intubate the patient may be severely restricted and in these cases it is invariably safer to move the casualty first.)

Inducing and paralysing a patient in a confined area is asking for trouble. A nasopharyngeal airway and rapid extraction is more appropriate. It is also worth noting that in a CBRN (Chemical, Biological, Radiological, Nuclear) environment most authorities advocate simple airway manoeuvres until the casualty has been removed from the hazard and decontaminated.

3.3.1.7 History

If possible some basic history should be sought with special reference to anaesthesia. The AMPLE history is acceptable (Box 3.6). If the patient is conscious, their name, date of birth and next of kin details allow for more effective administration in hospital.

Box 3.6: The AMPLE History
- **A**llergies
- **M**edications
- **P**ast Medical History
- **L**ast meal
- **E**vents leading to injury

3.3.2 *Prepare Equipment and Drugs*

The equipment required for intubation should have a standard configuration and everyone in the team should be familiar with it. It should be packed so that all items are easily accessible. Equipment bags based on the tool-roll principle can be effective for this purpose. These open out into a predictable configuration with individual items held securely in place. Items can be easily checked and are immediately at hand, and are unlikely to be left behind when withdrawing from the scene. Alternatively a "kit dump" can be prepared on a clean folded drape or clinical waste bag (Figs. 3.10 and 3.11). This has the advantage of being easily seen and avoided by other emergency service personnel.

3.3.2.1 PRSI Checklist (Appendix "PRSI Checklist")

Most airway equipment is single use, and it is generally advocated that it remains in original packaging until use. All equipment should be checked in the pre-RSI phase. The team does this together, with one calling out the list and the other checking the kit (Fig. 3.12). Laryngoscope handles should

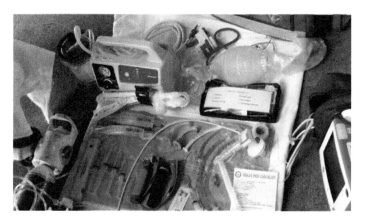

FIGURE 3.10 The equipment required to safely conduct PRSI

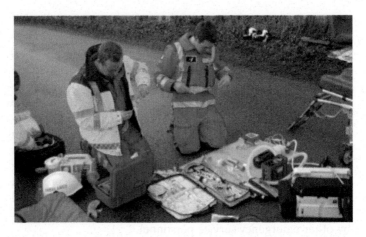

FIGURE 3.11 A pre-hospital team drawing up drugs and preparing an equipment dump

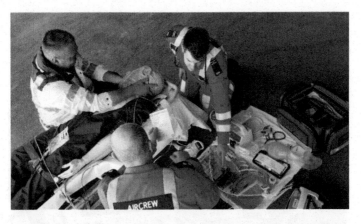

FIGURE 3.12 Challenge and response taking place using the checklist prior to PRSI

have working batteries and there should be two blades with functioning bulbs. An appropriately sized endotracheal tube (ETT) should be prepared: check the cuff does not leak, then fully deflate and lubricate it. An ETT a size smaller than estimated should always be easily accessible in case of unexpected difficulties. In patients with stridor or suspected airway oedema, an ETT 1–2 sizes smaller than normal should also be prepared.

A suitable bougie (tracheal tube introducer) must be available. A 10 mL syringe is required for inflating the ETT cuff, and tape or tie must be prepared for securing the ETT in position once placement is confirmed (or use a specifically designed tube holder).

Minimum monitoring standards are mandatory (Pulse oximeter, non-invasive blood pressure (NIBP), capnography and electrocardiogram (ECG)). In certain circumstances full monitoring may not be possible. A pulse oximeter may not function if the patient is cold or peripherally shutdown and even grossly assessing the colour of the patient (blue vs. pink) may be difficult in poor lighting. NIBP may need to be done manually by palpation or simply by ensuring the presence of a radial pulse. End-Tidal Carbon Dioxide ($ETCO_2$) is the gold standard for confirming tracheal intubation and is also important for monitoring ventilation during transport, particularly in head injured patients (See Chap. 6).

Sedative and paralysing agents should be prepared in standard concentrations and carefully labelled using standardised drug label stickers or permanent ink on the syringe barrel. The doses are then calculated appropriately for the patient's weight and condition (Appendix: Drug Dose, Weight & ETT Size Field Guide). Drugs and doses should then be cross-checked with another team member. Preparing essential drugs on a daily basis or using commercial or pharmacy pre-filled syringes may be an option. This reduces the risk of dilution and labelling errors on scene, and also offers the advantage of a shorter preparation time. Daily-prepared drugs can be wasteful and expensive if their use is infrequent.

Most neuromuscular blocking agents used in pre-hospital practice (e.g. Rocuronium, Suxamethonium) ideally require refrigerated storage. They degrade over time, and the rate of degradation increases with higher temperatures. Where such drugs are stored without refrigeration, organisations must have a system for wasting and replacing drugs that have not been used within the designated time period.

3.3.3   Positioning

During PRSI, 360° access to the patient is preferable. In addition, it is usually easier to perform laryngoscopy with the patient off the ground. If possible the patient should be on an ambulance trolley or elevated spinal board/scoop stretcher in preparation for induction. Having the trolley at knee height with team members kneeling is ideal, as this allows equipment and monitors to be left on the ground but within reach.

Kneeling to intubate whilst the patient is on a trolley is probably the best all round position. A trolley is not always immediately available however, and many pre-hospital intubations take place with the patient on the ground. Sitting back from the kneeling position onto the plantar flexed feet provides probably the most favoured way of intubating someone on the ground. To reduce strain on the neck, it is important to position the knees a few inches back from the patient's head, giving a better line of sight towards the larynx (Fig. 3.16).

An alternative to the 'kneeling back' position, is lying prone (Fig. 3.13a). This brings the intubator's eyes closer to the larynx, however it places the intubator at a mechanical disadvantage when applying a correct laryngoscopy technique (i.e. pulling 'up and away', with the laryngoscope handle at 45° to the ground). The prone position places emphasis on the anterior deltoid muscle and causes a tendency to lever back on the top teeth to improve the view, particularly in a more difficult intubation.

The seated position with legs either side of the patient's chest is another alternative (Fig. 3.13b). This provides a stable position with good mechanical advantage; it allows the stronger bicep muscle to be used and the elbow of the left arm can be supported against the left thigh if needed. It also requires less space at the head of the patient, however it can interfere with positioning of the equipment dump and moves the person providing MILS slightly further away from the patient.

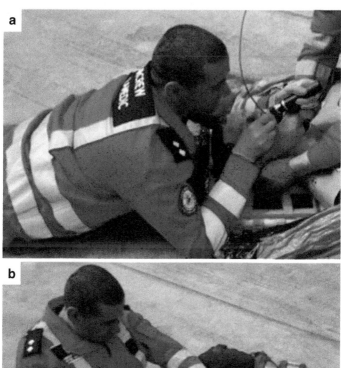

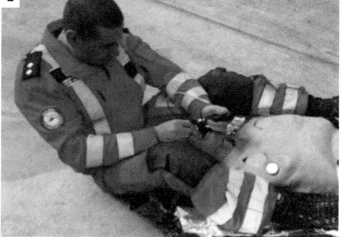

FIGURE 3.13 Alternative intubating positions (**a**) Lying prone, (**b**) Sitting

The trained assistant is ideally positioned facing the intubator on the side of the patient where IV access has been gained (it is slightly easier if this is on the patient's right so the

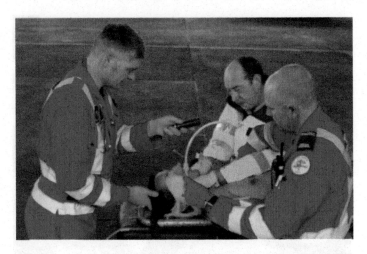

FIGURE 3.14 One assistant applies cricoid pressure and passes equipment whilst one assistant provides MILS

assistant can easily pass airway items into the right hand of the intubator). The kit dump is placed between the intubator and assistant so that both are able to reach kit if required. If on the right side of the patient, the assistant provides cricoid pressure with the right hand and passes equipment with the left and vice versa (Fig. 3.14). Given the potential for inappropriately applied cricoid pressure to be either ineffective or to impede intubation, it is not advisable to ask others with little or no experience of the technique to take on this role.

If IV access is in the arm, either the intubator or the assistant should then be able to reach the cannula and administer drugs. It may be preferable (or necessary if only tibial IO access is available) for an additional person to administer drugs. Instructions regarding drug doses must be explicit and understood prior to commencing PRSI. This extra person can also be used to continuously palpate the radial pulse during induction, in order to promptly detect the requirement for a vasopressor/inotrope/fluid. Without this additional person, it is easy for the intubator and assistant to become focused on the airway and fail to notice, and respond promptly to a drop in blood pressure.

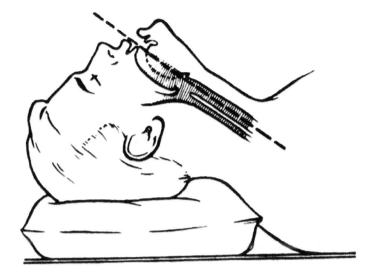

FIGURE 3.15 'Sniffing the morning air' position with neck flexed and head extended

The monitor is placed so that both the intubator and assistant can see it. This usually means next to the kit dump, but further away from the patient. If the patient is on a trolley, this may require the monitor to be tilted back to get a clear view of the screen.

The "sniffing the morning air" position (Fig. 3.15); with the neck flexed and head extended, is the ideal intubating position, however this is not appropriate if there is a possibility of cervical spine injury. If manual in-line stabilisation (MILS) of the cervical spine is required, it is carried out from the opposite side to the trained assistant. If any task is to be devolved to a non-team member, it is MILS, as it is relatively easy to instruct another member of the emergency services to undertake this role.

It may be useful to position a bystander at the foot of the casualty in order to tilt the patient head down should the oropharynx fill with vomit or blood during induction. A functioning high pressure, high volume suction unit should always be immediately to hand with a manual unit in reserve.

3.3.4   Protection

3.3.4.1   Cervical Spine Injury

A cervical spine injury will have been sustained by 2.4 % of blunt trauma victims (Crosby 2006). If the GCS is <8 this figure increases to 10.2 %. The indications for PHA (e.g. respiratory compromise, reduced GCS etc.), will preclude pre-hospital clearance of the cervical spine as the patient will either not be fully conscious or will have a distracting injury. Therefore, if the mechanism of injury is consistent with a cervical spine injury, MILS should be initiated.

Manual In-Line Stabilisation (MILS)

When three or more team members are present, MILS is best performed from the opposite site of the casualty to the assistant, approaching over the front of the chest (Fig. 3.16). MILS can alternatively be applied from above the patient's head, on either side of the intubator, but this involves sharing a lim-

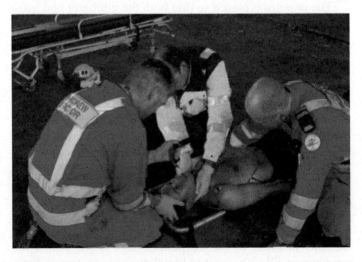

FIGURE 3.16 MILS can be performed over the chest from the opposite side to the assistant

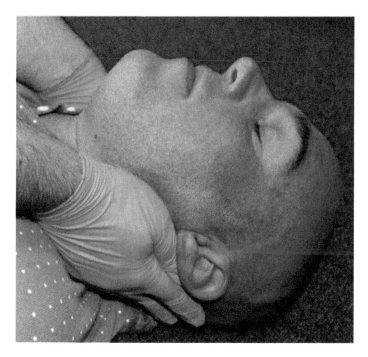

FIGURE 3.17 Correct MILS hand position with thumbs applying pressure down on mastoid processes behind the ears leaving the jaw free to move during laryngoscopy

ited space and can impede the intubation process. The aim of MILS is to oppose the forces generated by laryngoscopy and is achieved by firmly holding down the patient's mastoid processes (Fig. 3.17). This affords a good mechanical advantage to oppose movement during laryngoscopy and reduces the degree of head extension by 50 % (Hasting and Wood 1994). When only two team members are in attendance a "careful" intubation may be all that is possible. Intubating whilst attempting to stabilise the head between the knees in a kneeling position is possible, but this requires an awkward leaning back position to view the larynx, which is a strain in a difficult intubation.

If the patient is already immobilised with a hard collar and head blocks, these should be removed (the collar may simply be opened or the front part removed) and replaced by MILS. Full spinal immobilisation is independently associated with an increased risk of difficult intubation (Heath 1994). Removing the collar significantly improves mouth opening (Goutcher and Lochead 2005), but MILS will still impede a view at laryngoscopy compared to the optimum position. Nolan reported a reduced view in 45 % of "normal" elective patients, with no view of the larynx at all in 22 % (Nolan and Wilson 1993). Reassuringly, although five patients were unable to be intubated directly, all were intubated success-fully with the use of a bougie. A bougie is superior to a mal-leable stylet to aid intubation (Gataure et al. 1996; Noguchi et al. 2003), and should be used routinely in PRSI to increase intubation success. Performing a RSI with MILS using a gum elastic bougie is very unlikely to cause further cervical spine movement (Crosby 2006). However, always remember: Failure to oxygenate may kill the patient; moving the neck will probably not.

3.3.4.2   Cricoid Pressure

This is a technique used in anaesthesia to decrease the risk of aspiration during induction. The application of cricoid pressure is also known as Sellick's manoeuvre after the anaesthetist who first described it in 1961 (Sellick 1961). During induction the tone of the upper oesophageal sphinc-ter is reduced and the airway reflexes lost. This means that gastric contents may passively move up the oesophagus, into the oropharynx and soil the airway. The application of cricoid pressure compensates for this loss of tone by compressing the proximal oesophageal lumen between the cricoid cartilage and the cervical vertebrae.

The cricoid cartilage is chosen, as it is the only part of the airway that consists of a complete ring of cartilage (Fig. 3.18). The thyroid cartilage and tracheal rings have only soft tissue posteriorly and are ineffective at compressing the oesophagus.

Cricoid pressure is a 3-finger technique. Sellick described the manoeuvre as follows: "Before induction the cricoid is

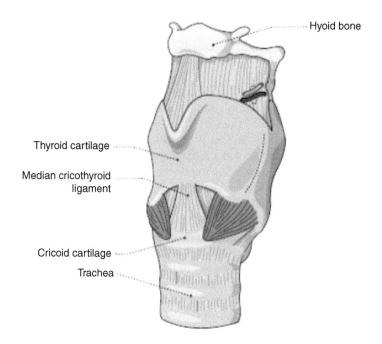

Hyoid bone

Thyroid cartilage

Median cricothyroid ligament

Cricoid cartilage

Trachea

FIGURE 3.18 Upper airway anatomy

palpated and lightly held between the thumb and second finger; as anaesthesia begins, pressure is exerted on the cricoid cartilage mainly by the index finger."

Sellick reported the technique as a 1-handed manoeuvre. Some groups have advocated the use of a 2-handed technique, with the second hand providing counter pressure behind the neck. This technique may have utility as when anterior force is applied, neck flexion is possible. This may potentially exacerbate a cervical spine injury. It appears, however, that when the correct force is used in the correct direction, there is no clear additional advantage to the provision of posterior neck support (Cook 1996; Vanner et al. 1997). Therefore, in both the hospital and pre-hospital environment a 1-handed technique is usual. This technique has the added advantage of allowing the assistant to deliver cricoid pressure *and* pass equipment during intubation.

It has been shown that a force of 30 N is necessary to achieve oesophageal occlusion and prevent regurgitation (Vanner and Asai 1999). This pressure is described as "firm pressure" or that required to cause pain when applied to the bridge of the nose.

Smith and Dejoy (2001) recommended applying 10 N of force prior to induction and then 30 N when the patient loses consciousness. More than 20 N of force is uncomfortable and can cause retching, so it is preferable to simply position the fingers over the cricoid cartilage prior to induction rather than accidentally applying excessive pressure too early.

Correctly applied cricoid pressure may enhance the laryngoscopic view and facilitate intubation in some patients. More likely, it will impede the view at laryngoscopy (Haslam et al. 2005). Excessive force (>40 N) may lead to distortion of the upper airway. This may make both intubation more difficult, and impede mask ventilation in the event of a failed intubation. Cricoid pressure should be applied directly backwards, but it is easy to accidentally apply pressure to either the left or right (usually the opposite side to the person applying the pressure). The intubator should be aware of these potential problems and be prepared to move the hand of the assistant in an attempt to visualise the larynx. The intubator should have a low threshold for requesting reduction or even removal of cricoid pressure if they consider that their view is being impeded by its application.

In addition to the above problems, inadequate pressure may be ineffective and still allow regurgitation. Similarly, pressure applied in the wrong place, (e.g. thyroid cartilage) will not be effective either. Given the potential for problems, it is important that the assistant is trained and proficient in this technique, particularly when the intubator is relatively inexperienced. It is well recognised that even experienced anaesthetic assistants may have a poor technique if not recently practised. However, this can be easily improved by a very short period of simple retraining (May and Trethewy 2007; Owen et al. 2002). Experience in delivering the correct pressure can be achieved using mechanical simulators, kitchen scales or even a 50 mL syringe (compressing the plunger on a capped off, air-filled 50 mL syringe to 33 mL approximates to 30 N) (Flucker et al. 2000; Herman et al. 1996).

If passive regurgitation occurs, pressure should be increased and the oropharynx suctioned immediately. Conversely, cricoid pressure should actually be released if active vomiting occurs at induction. This may occur before any/sufficient induction agent has been given, and can sometimes be provoked by excessive and early cricoid pressure. In this case the continued application of force to the cricoid can result in oesophageal rupture.

Cricoid pressure should be applied as the patient loses consciousness or ceases respiratory effort (if already unconscious). Ideally it should not be released before the endotracheal tube has been placed, the cuff inflated, and its position confirmed. The caveat to this is that removal may be requested to improve the view at laryngoscopy, as described above. It is permissible to gently ventilate the lungs with cricoid pressure in situ, should it be necessary to maintain adequate oxygenation prior to laryngoscopy, as this should reduce gas entering and distending the stomach.

In a prospective observational study of 402 patients, Harris et al. (2010) reported on the effects of cricoid pressure and laryngeal manipulation in a UK HEMS service. They compared the effect on laryngoscopic view of three laryngeal manoeuvres; release of cricoid pressure, BURP or laryngeal manipulation. These manoeuvres were used during 61 intubations when the intubator was either unable to see the cords or to pass the bougie through the cords. The laryngoscopic view was improved by at least one Cormack-Lehane grade with release of cricoid pressure in 11 of 22 patients (50 %), with laryngeal manipulation in 15 of 25 patients (60 %), and with BURP in 9 of 14 patients (64 %). No manoeuvre made the view worse. Release of cricoid pressure was followed by regurgitation in two patients, both of whom had received prolonged BVM ventilation.

Given the evidence of pre-hospital aspiration described earlier, the benefit of cricoid pressure is not proven. It is most likely to be beneficial in those who have not yet lost laryngeal reflexes (i.e., GCS >8), in order to reduce aspiration risk when they relax under anaesthesia. To avoid confusion, it is advisable to use cricoid pressure for every PRSI, but to be aware of the limited evidence and have a low threshold for adjusting/releasing it when faced with a difficult intubation.

3.4   Premedication

Pretreatment with a drug (before giving the induction agent) is usually aimed at obtunding the sympathetic response to laryngoscopy whilst allowing a reduced dose of induction agent to be used to achieve the same end result. The pretreatment drugs are therefore ideally more cardiostable than the induction agents. Examples of drugs used for pretreatment include Fentanyl and Alfentanil.

3.5   Paralyse and Sedate

The induction phase should only be commenced when all preparation is complete. Other than in peri-arrest situations, the team should have already run through the PRSI checklist to ensure that nothing has been missed.

PRSI should then begin with the administration of an induction agent, (preceded by pretreatment if appropriate). The dose of the induction drug should be adjusted to account for level of consciousness, other drugs already given/taken, volume status, blood pressure and ICP. Many induction agents cause hypotension. This hypotension may result from peripheral vasodilatation, a reduction in cardiac contractility or a reduction in intrinsic sympathetic tone. Hypotension is most marked in hypovolaemic patients but may not be immediately obvious after intubation due to the sympathetic response to laryngoscopy. Ketamine is an exception to this rule, and blood pressure is usually maintained due to its action on the sympathetic nervous system.

Hypotension is a predictable side effect, and vigilance with prompt management is essential. Ideally one person should be tasked to monitor the radial pulse both during and after induction. Prophylactic treatment may be considered in certain situations, with a fluid bolus being administered prior to induction. A vasopressor or inotrope should be on hand to manage episodes of hypotension resistant to fluid therapy.

Loss of consciousness (e.g. loss of eyelash reflex or loss of verbal response) is normally assured prior to administration of the muscle relaxant (paralysing agent). Suxamethonium 1.5 mg/kg was traditionally used because of its rapid onset, but is associated with many side effects (Box 3.7). It is frequently cited that a benefit of Suxamethonium over other muscle relaxants is its short duration of action. The suggestion was that in the event of failed intubation the patient would recommence spontaneous respiration and therefore avoid critical hypoxia. In reality, critical desaturation is likely to occur prior to muscular activity returning, so assisted ventilation will be required (Benumof et al. 1997). As it is easier to ventilate a fully relaxed patient in the event of failed intubation, this argument does not hold. More significantly, the vast majority of patients undergoing PRSI are not suitable to be safely managed 'awake'. Continued anaesthesia and paralysis with an alternative form of advanced airway would be preferable. Rocuronium 1.2 mg/kg has a slightly increased onset time compared to Suxamethonium, but many fewer side effects (although there is still an incidence of anaphylaxis) (see Chap. 6). For these reasons, Rocuronium is now widely used in PHA throughout the UK.

The paralysing agent should always be followed by a flush to ensure the drug reaches its point of action in as short a time as possible. The onset of paralysis may be prolonged in a patient with a low cardiac output state. When using Suxamethonium its onset is usually heralded by fasciculations but these are not always seen. Non-depolarising muscle relaxants, such as Rocuronium, do not generate fasciculations. As a guide, laryngoscopy should be attempted only when the mouth opens freely. This equates well to cord paralysis.

Box 3.7: Side Effects of Suxamethonium
- Anaphylaxis
- Malignant hyperthermia (including masseter spasm)
- Hyperkalaemia (>24 h after burns or spinal injury)
- Severe muscle pains

3.6   Passage of Tube

The aim is to be swift but not rushed. The whole process should take no more than 1 min.

The vocal cords are attached anteriorly to the thyroid cartilage and posteriorly to the arytenoid cartilages (Figs. 3.18 and 3.19). The view is described by the Cormack and Lehane classification (Fig. 3.20). A modification divides grade 2 into:

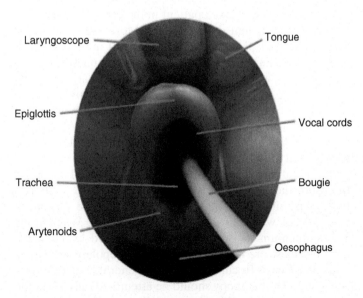

FIGURE 3.19 View at laryngoscopy (manikin)

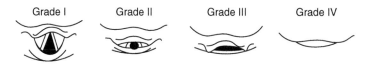

FIGURE 3.20 Cormack and Lehane intubation grade (Reproduced with kind permission Anaesthesia UK Website)

grade 2a: part of the vocal cords are seen and 2b: only the arytenoids seen. This should be recorded along with additional equipment required (e.g., McCoy blade) and handed over to other medical personnel, indicating the difficulty or otherwise of intubation.

A poor view may be improved by *Backward Upward* (pushing an anterior larynx backwards and then up towards the laryngoscope) *Rightward* (as the laryngoscope is coming in from the right side of the mouth/tongue) *Pressure* (BURP) on the thyroid and cricoid cartilages together.

3.6.1 *Laryngoscope*

A Macintosh size 3 laryngoscope is suitable for most adults and is easier to insert than a size 4 when mouth opening is limited. A size 4 may be required in patients with a large jaw. Care should be taken not to insert a size 4 too far initially as it is easy to pass the larynx and reach the oesophagus which can be difficult to recognise for the inexperienced.

A McCoy blade, which has a flexible tip, (Fig. 6.6) has been shown to significantly improve the view at laryngoscopy when the neck is immobilised (Gabbott 1996). There is therefore an argument for using one routinely in the pre-hospital environment. Unfortunately they are not currently available in disposable form and require appropriate cleaning between patients. Many practitioners are also not experienced in the technique required to use a McCoy laryngoscope.

Other laryngoscope devices including indirect laryngoscopes (e.g. Airtraq®) (Fig. 6.7) and video laryngoscopes (e.g. Glidescope®) (Fig. 6.8), have been demonstrated to improve laryngoscopic view and intubation success rate in patients with cervical spine immobilisation or other predicted 'difficult' airways in the hospital setting (Maharaj et al. 2007; Malik et al. 2009; McElwain and Laffey 2011). These have great potential to be useful airway devices in the pre-hospital setting, but as yet evidence for their use is limited. Contamination (such as blood and vomit) in the airways of pre-hospital patients, poses a significant challenge to the optical arrangements of such laryngoscopes (Trimmel et al. 2011), and personnel should have experience and regular training with these devices before attempting to use them for PRSI.

3.6.2 Bougie

A gum elastic bougie (or disposable tracheal introducer of a similar design) should be used electively in all PRSIs due to the increased incidence of difficult intubation (Figs. 3.21 and 3.22). When only the arytenoids are visible, by using a bougie, correct placement should still be relatively straightforward. Even when only the epiglottis is seen, this can be used as a landmark to guide the blind placement of a bougie.

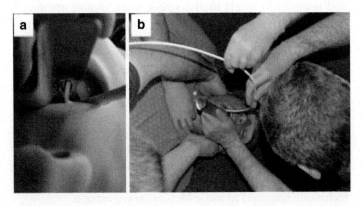

FIGURE 3.21 (a) A view of the bougie passing between the cords with tip angled anteriorly. (b) The intubator passing a bougie through the vocal cords before an ETT is railroaded over the top

The "click" of the tip of the bougie passing over the tracheal cartilages may be felt, confirming correct placement. Alternatively, resistance will occur as the bougie reaches the carina or bronchi, whereas it will generally pass unhindered down the length of the oesophagus. The latter technique can only be used if the bougie is used independently then the ETT railroaded over afterwards by the assistant (rather than preloading the ETT on the bougie). Preloading the ETT also requires the bougie to be held firmly below the tip of the ETT to allow control of the tip. This is best understood by practise on a manikin.

A bougie needs to be either stored straight or gently curved with the angled tip on the *inside* of the curve. A bent or misshapen bougie can be very difficult to use. In hot temperatures, a gum elastic bougie can become very soft and unusable; storing in a cool box may be necessary to maintain some rigidity. A bougie made of an alternative material may therefore be preferable in a hot environment.

The ETT will sometimes be held up as the tip catches on the vocal cords. This can be resolved by rotating the ETT anticlockwise 90° in the majority of cases. Occasionally cricoid pressure will need to be released.

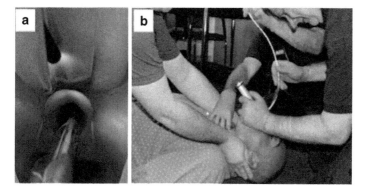

FIGURE 3.22 (**a**) An ETT being passed over a bougie with the laryngoscope in the vallecula, (**b**) The bougie is held still by the assistant while the intubator railroads the ETT through the vocal cords

The incidence of complications markedly increases after two failed attempts at passing an endotracheal tube (Mort 2004). For this reason, after two attempts the failed intubation drill is followed. It is only worth attempting intubation for a second time if something is going to be changed for the second attempt i.e. position of the patient, different size blade, different laryngoscope type (e.g. McCoy, Airtraq™). Repeating exactly the same manoeuvre will likely give the same view and delay the establishment of adequate oxygenation/ventilation by another means. Ventilation should be carried out between attempts if required to maintain SpO_2 above 92 %.

3.6.3   Plan A and Plan B

When embarking on an RSI it is essential to be clear not only about your primary objective but also to have a prepared fallback position should things go wrong (Box 3.8). As previously mentioned, in the pre-hospital environment, when faced with a failed intubation, waking the patient up is unlikely to be clinically appropriate.

Box 3.8: Planning for PRSI
- *Plan A* – A successful rapid sequence intubation
- *Plan B* – A contingency for "failed intubation"

3.6.4   Failed Intubation Drill (Appendix "Failed Intubation Protocol")

In the event of a failure to intubate during PRSI a well-rehearsed drill should increase the likelihood of a good outcome. The intubator should rapidly recognise that the situation requires the implementation of the "Failed Intubation Drill" and should clearly declare this to the assistant. The assistant should then immediately release cricoid pressure and pass the LMA (Appendix "Use of the Laryngeal Mask Airway") or other supraglottic airway device (SAD). If a LMA is used there are advantages to using one that allows higher ventilation pressures to be delivered e.g. Proseal™ LMA (Fig. A.3). The assistant should then immediately prepare the surgical cricothyroidotomy kit in case this is required. If ventilation is unsuccessful with the rescue device, ventilation with a BVM and oropharyngeal airway should be attempted, whilst the most experienced team member performs a surgical cricothyroidotomy (Appendix "Emergency Cricothyroidotomy"). When Suxamethonium is the muscle relaxant used, it may be beginning to wear off. A second dose should be avoided, as it can induce a profound bradycardia; a non-depolarising muscle relaxant, such as Rocuronium, should be used instead.

3.7 Post Intubation

3.7.1 Confirmation of Placement

Unrecognised oesophageal intubation is a preventable and catastrophic complication of PRSI. The gold standard for ensuring correct ETT positioning is the presence of $ETCO_2$ using capnography (See Chap. 6).

Other methods are used to confirm correct placement, but can be misleading and are not infallible. These include:

Visual Confirmation: The ETT may be seen to pass through the cords. Unfortunately the view is often not ideal, and when railroading the tube, any view one had of the larynx, may be blocked by the passing tube.

Auscultation: Listening (in both axillae) with a stethoscope may confirm air entry in the lungs. It will also confirm bilateral ventilation and confirm that the tube has not been inserted too far i.e., into the right main bronchus. Unfortunately breath sounds can be difficult to hear in some patients (e.g., obese, emphysema) and this is often exacerbated in the pre-hospital environment due to external noise.

Look and Feel: Chest movement may be seen or felt with hands placed on the chest. This is not very reliable.

Oesophageal Detector: These are commercial devices based on the "Wee oesophageal detector." They are essentially large syringes that are attached to the ETT, and an attempt is made to rapidly withdraw air. If the tube is in the trachea, this is easy to do, if in the oesophagus, resistance is felt due to collapse of the compliant walls of the oesophagus. This technique can be reassuring in patients in cardiac arrest when minimal carbon dioxide is being produced and this cannot be detected convincingly by any of the methods described earlier. An oesophageal detector is accurate in adult patients, however false positives can occur in very obese patients and children due to collapse of the trachea.

References

American Society of Anesthesiologists. Practice guidelines for management of the difficult airway: a report by the American Society for Anesthesiologists Task Force on Management of the Difficult Airway. Anesthesiology. 1993;78:597–602.

American Society of Anesthesiologists. Practice guidelines for management of the difficult airway: an updated report by The American Society of Anesthesiologists Task Force on Management of the Difficult Airway. Anesthesiology. 2013;118(2):251–70.

Barnard EBG, Moy RJ, Kehoe AD, et al. Rapid sequence induction of anesthesia via the intraosseous route: a prospective observational study. Emerg Med J. 2014. [published online first: doi:10.1136/emermed-2014-203740].

Benumof JL, Dagg R, Benumof R. Critical hemoglobin desaturation will occur before a return to an unparalyzed state following 1 mg/kg intravenous succinylcholine. Anesthesiology. 1997;87: 979–82.

Brohi K, Cohen MJ, Davenport RA. Acute coagulopathy of trauma: mechanism, identification and effect. Curr Opin Crit Care. 2007;13: 680–5.

Breckwoldt J, Klemstein S, Brunne B, et al. Difficult prehospital endotracheal intubation – predisposing factors in a physician based EMS. Resuscitation. 2011;82:1519–24.

Cook TM. Cricoid pressure: are two hands better than one. Anaesthesia. 1996;51:365–8.

Cooper BR, Mahoney P, Hodgetts TJ, Mellor A. Intra-osseous access (EZ-IO®) for resuscitation: UK military combat experience. J R Army Med Corps. 2007;153:314–6.

Crosby ED. Airway management in adults after cervical spine trauma. Anesthesiology. 2006;104:1293–318.

Fakhry SM, et al. Prehospital rapid sequence intubation for head trauma: conditions for a successful program. J Trauma. 2006;60:997–1001.

Flucker CJ, Hart E, Weisz M, et al. The 50 millilitre syringe as an inexpensive training aid in the application of cricoid pressure. Eur J Anaesthesiol. 2000;17:443–7.

Gabbott DA. Laryngoscopy using the McCoy laryngoscope after application of a cervical collar. Anaesthesia. 1996;51:812–4.

Gataure PS, Vaughan RS, Latto IP. Simulated difficult intubation. Comparison of the gum elastic bougie and the stylet. Anaesthesia. 1996;51:935–8.

Goutcher CM, Lochead V. Reduction in mouth opening with semi-rigid cervical collars. Br J Anaesth. 2005;95:344–8.

Greaves I, Porter KM, Ryan JM, editors. Shock. In: Trauma care manual. London: Arnold; 2000. p. 78–9.

Harris T, Ellis DY, Foster L, Lockey D. Cricoid pressure and laryngeal manipulation in 402 pre-hospital emergency anaesthetics: Essential safety measure or a hindrance to rapid safe intubation? Resuscitation. 2010;81:810–6.

Haslam N, Parker L, Duggan JE. Effect of cricoid pressure on the view at laryngoscopy. Anaesthesia. 2005;60:41–7.

Hasting RH, Wood PR. Head extension and laryngeal view during laryngoscopy with cervical spine immobilization maneuvers. Anesthesiology. 1994;80:825–31.

Heath KJ. The effect of laryngoscopy on different cervical spine immobilization techniques. Anaesthesia. 1994;49:843–5.

Herman NL, Carter B, Van Decar TK. Cricoid pressure: teaching the recommended level. Anesth Analg. 1996;83:859–63.

Lane S, Saunders D, Schofield A, et al. A prospective randomised controlled trial comparing the efficacy of preoxygenation in the 20 degrees head-up vs supine position. Anaesthesia. 2005;20:1064–7.

Lockey D, Crewdson K, Weaver A, Davies G. Observational study of the success rates of intubation and failed intubation airway rescue techniques in 7256 attempted intubations of trauma patients by pre-hospital physicians. Br J Anaes. 2014;113(2): 220–5.

Lockey DJ, Avery P, Harris T, et al. A prospective study of physician pre-hospital anaesthesia in trauma patients: oesophageal intubation, gross airway contamination and the 'quick look' airway assessment. BMC Anesthesiol. 2013;13:21.

Maharaj CH, Buckley E, Harte BH, Laffey JG. Endotracheal intubation in patients with cervical spine immobilization: a comparison of macintosh and airtraq laryngoscopes. Anesthesiology. 2007;107:53–9.

Malik MA, Subramaniam R, Maharaj CH, Harte BH, Laffey JG. Randomized controlled trial of the Pentax AWS®, Glidescope® and Macintosh laryngoscopes in predicted difficult intubations. Br J Anaesth. 2009;103(5):761–8.

May P, Trethewy C. Practice makes perfect? Evaluation of cricoid pressure task training for use within the algorithm for rapid sequence induction in critical care. Emerg Med Australas. 2007;19:207–12.

McElwain J, Laffey JG. Comparison of the C-MAC®, Airtraq®, and Macintosh laryngoscopes in patients undergoing tracheal intubation with cervical spine immobilization. Br J Anaesth. 2011;107(2):258–64.

Mills PJ, Baptiste J, Preston J, Barnas GM. Manual resuscitators and spontaneous ventilation – an evaluation. Crit Care Med. 1991;19:1425–31.

Mort TC. Emergency tracheal intubation; complications associated with repeated larynogoscopic attempts. Anesth Analg. 2004;99:607–13.

Murray GD, et al. Multivariable prognostic analysis in traumatic brain injury: results from the IMPACT study. J Neurotrauma. 2007;24:329–37.

Nimmagadda U, Salem MR, Joseph NJ, et al. Efficacy of preoxygenation with tidal volume breathing. Comparison of breathing systems. Anesthesiology. 2000;93:693–8.

Noguchi T, Koga K, Shiga Y, Shigematsu A. The gum elastic bougie eases tracheal intubation while applying cricoid pressure compared to a stylet. Can J Anaesth. 2003;50:712–7.

Nolan JP, Wilson ME. Orotracheal intubation in patients with potential cervical spine injuries. An indication for the gum elastic bougie. Anaesthesia. 1993;48:630–3.

Owen H, Follows V, Reynolds KJ, et al. Learning to apply effective cricoid pressure using a part task trainer. Anaesthesia. 2002;57:1098–101.

Perel P, Roberts I, Ker K. Colloids versus crystalloids for fluid resuscitation in critically ill patients (Review). Cochrane Database Syst Rev. 2013;1. doi: 10.1002/14651858.CD000567.pub6

Ramkumar V, Umesh G, Philip FA. Preoxygenation with 20° head-up tilt provides longer duration of non-hypoxic apnea than conventional preoxygenation in non-obese healthy adults. J Anesth. 2011;25:189–94.

Sellick BA. Cricoid pressure to control regurgitation of stomach contents during induction of anaesthesia. Lancet. 1961;2:404–5.

Smith C, Dejoy SJ. New equipment and techniques for airway management in trauma. Curr Opin Anaesthesiol. 2001;14:197–209.

Spahn DR, Bouillon B, Cerny V, et al. Management of bleeding and coagulopathy following major trauma: an updated European guideline. Crit Care. 2013;17:R76.

Trimmel H, Kreutziger J, Fertsak G, Fitzka R, Dittrich M, Voelckel WG. Use of the Airtraq laryngoscope for emergency intubation in the prehospital setting: a randomized control trial. Crit Care Med. 2011;39(3):489–93.

Vanner RG, Asai T. Safe use of cricoid pressure. Anaesthesia. 1999;54:1–3.

Vanner RG, Clarke P, Moore WJ, Raftery S. The effect of cricoid pressure and neck support on the view at laryngoscopy. Anaesthesia. 1997;52:896–900.

Wang HE, Davis DP, Wayne MA, Delbridge T. Prehospital rapid-sequence intubation-what does the evidence show? Prehosp Emerg Care. 2004;8:366–77.

Weingart SD, Levitan RM. Preoxygenation and prevention of desaturation during emergency airway management. Ann Emerg Med. 2012;59(3):165–75.

Weingart SD, Trueger NS, Wong N, et al. Delayed sequence intubation: a prospective observational study. Ann Emerg Med. 2015;65(4):349–55.

Wimalasena YH, Corfield AR, Hearns S. Comparison of factors associated with desaturation in prehospital emergency anaesthesia in primary and secondary retrieval. Emerg Med J. 2014. [published online first: doi:10.1136/emermed-2013-202928].

Wimalasena YH, Burns B, Reid C, et al. Apneic oxygenation was associated with decreased desaturation rates during rapid sequence intubation by an Australian Helicopter Emergency Medicine Service. Ann Emerg Med. 2015;65(4):371–6.

Xeropotamos NS, Coats TJ, Wilson AW. Prehospital surgical airway management: 1 year's experience from the Helicopter Emergency Medical Service. Injury. 1993;24:222–4.

Chapter 4
Crew Resource Management (CRM)

By the end of this chapter you will be able to:

- Define Crew Resource Management, Human Factors and Non-Technical Skills
- Understand the importance of Crew Resource Management in the pre-hospital environment
- Discuss the component factors of Crew Resource Management in pre-hospital anaesthetic practice

Pre-hospital anaesthesia (PHA) is a potentially high-risk procedure in a challenging environment. A successful outcome relies on dynamic interaction between several members of a multidisciplinary team. The skills involved can be divided into those of a technical nature, such as laryngoscopy, and those of a non-technical nature, such as teamwork and communication. These latter skills arguably play a larger part in determining the safe and successful completion of the procedure, than the individual technical skills of team-members.

Errors are an inevitable part of complex systems with human involvement, and can lead to adverse events. The 'Swiss

T. Lowes et al., *Pre-Hospital Anesthesia Handbook*,
DOI 10.1007/978-3-319-23090-0_4,
© Springer-Verlag London 2016

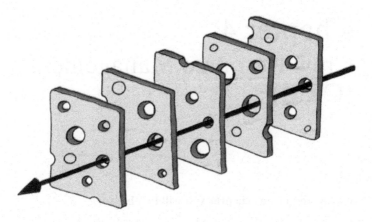

FIGURE 4.1 Reason's Swiss cheese model (Reason 2000)

Cheese Model' (Fig. 4.1) demonstrates that, occasionally, the holes in several slices of cheese can line up perfectly to allow an error to pass through without being blocked. Adverse incidents are generally the result of a sequence of coincidental circumstances, misjudgements and technical errors. These often occur on a background of latent flaws in a system, which reduce the chance for prevention.

The aviation industry has for many years recognised that training in non-technical skills reduces errors and improves safety. Crew (previously Cockpit) Resource Management training originated from a NASA workshop in 1979 (Cooper et al 1980), and has been embedded within the culture of the aviation industry for over three decades. In simple terms, CRM is the ability to make best use of all available personnel and resources. This requires the use of cognitive, social and personal skills that complement the technical skills required to fly. They are the 'Non-Technical Skills' (Box 4.1) and the 'Human Factors' that can result in catastrophic outcomes when they are lacking from a team.

Box 4.1: Non-Technical Skills
- Situational Awareness
- Teamwork
- Leadership
- Communication
- Decision-Making
- Task Management (Prioritising)

Individuals are more likely to demonstrate these qualities if they have been trained and work in an organisation that provides the culture, working environment, processes, and equipment to support good CRM.

Assurance of competency in these non-technical skills is a component of licensing and revalidation for Pilots. Many comparisons can be drawn between the highly complex system within an aeroplane cockpit, and the multiple steps and interactions required to plan, prepare and undertake medical interventions (such as PHA) in a high-pressure environment. The concepts of CRM are sometimes referred to as Team Resource Management (TRM), and this is the term used in the current PHEM curriculum. This term appears to have been originally used by the European Organisation for the Safety of Air Navigation (1996) in a document relating to enhanced teamwork for Air Traffic Management staff and is now sometimes used synonymously with CRM.

4.1 Situational Awareness

Situational awareness refers to an individual's awareness of their immediate environment along with potential external influences, and the understanding and analysis of this to predict future events. Box 4.2 displays the three-stage model of situational awareness by Endsley (2001), along with examples of how failures in situational awareness can occur at each stage.

Box 4.2: Endsley's Three-Stage Model of Situational Awareness

Level 1	Perception – of environmental elements (Failure to correctly perceive the situation)
Example	You attend a Road Traffic Collision (RTC) where a car has gone off the road into a hedge. There is an injured driver and injured front seat passenger. You fail to notice the large impact on the front right of the car and external 'bulls-eye' on the window. You therefore do not think to look for the badly injured motorcyclist 100 m further down the road in a ditch
Level 2	Comprehension – of relevant information and derivation of meaning (Failure to comprehend the situation)
Example	Attending the same RTC you note the front-right impact and presume the car may have hit either another car or perhaps the gatepost next to the hedge, before reaching its final position. You note the damaged windscreen but presume this is from the driver. You fail to think that the damage must be external as the driver was wearing a seatbelt and he has only minor facial injuries with a deflated airbag in front of him.
Level 3	Projection – of future status (Failure to project the situation into the future)

(continued)

Box 4.2 (continued)

Example | Attending the same RTC you quickly assess the driver and front seat passenger. You note that the driver has minor injuries, but the passenger is shocked. You suspect he has a ruptured spleen and fractured femur, and is likely to require emergency surgery at the major trauma centre. The police officer and paramedic went to look for a possible third patient after you noted the external damage to the car, and inform you of a male motorcyclist with a head injury and reduced GCS. At this point you fail to think ahead and do not call for a second ambulance. Fifteen minutes later, after assessing and anaesthetising the motorcyclist you realise that you now have two patients requiring transfer to the major trauma centre and request assistance. Unfortunately by now the nearest ambulance is 15 miles further away attending another patient.

Lack of situational awareness may lead to poor decision-making and adverse events. A brief moment of assessment of the wider scene immediately on arrival is time well spent. Distractions must be avoided; this includes being drawn into the management of an individual patient before confirming the number of casualties and prioritising treatment. The clinician must gain 'control' of the scene, and an appreciation of the hazards of their working environment, as soon as possible.

Assimilating the relevant information, in a short period of time, is an essential skill of the experienced pre-hospital practitioner. In addition to the patient's history and current condition, the mechanism of injury, available personnel and equipment, along with weather and time of day, all require consideration. Various multiagency staff (such as fire, police and ambulance crews) can be integral to the team effort, but co-ordination of effort is required. Bystanders may be helpful in remote locations, but may require management to prevent them posing further risk.

4.2   Bandwidth and Stressors

The concept of 'Bandwidth' refers to an individual only being able to handle and process a certain amount of information at any one time. This varies from person to person. Those who become very task-focused and have limited peripheral vision (i.e., an inability to take on information outside their immediate focus) are described as having a 'narrowed bandwidth'. Psychological stressors and physiological distractions (being hot/cold/hungry etc.), limit information input and processing, and 'narrow' the bandwidth further. The Federal Aviation Authority's I'M SAFE checklist (2015) is a useful tool for recognition of physiological and psychological stressors (Elimination is often added to the E as a powerful physiological distraction) (Fig. 4.2) . In small teams that rely on all members performing well, this checklist can be used to pick up issues before the team starts their shift.

When 'overloaded' an individual may ignore further input, and not hear or see information presented to him/her. This can be an issue when fixation on a particular task, such as a difficult intubation, is completely occupying the available bandwidth of the individual performing that task. When this is anticipated, safety can be maintained by 'offloading' tasks, such as overall scene safety, bystander control, or monitoring blood pressure, to other members of the multi-agency pre-hospital team. Distribution of tasks allows the collective bandwidth of all individuals within the team to be utilised.

4.3   Teamwork and Leadership

Distribution of workload across members of a team and a collaborative approach, allows a complex task such as PHA to be achieved in a safe and timely manner. An effective team needs a shared purpose, an effective leader and supportive

I'M SAFE Checklist

Illness – Do I have any symptoms?

Medication – Have I been taking medication or drugs?

Stress – Am I under psychological pressure or worried about finance/health/family?

Alcohol – Have I been drinking within 8/24hrs?

Fatigue – Am I tired/inadequately rested?

Eating – Am I adequately nourished?

FIGURE 4.2 I'm safe checklist

team members. Too many leaders can be a hindrance; a team requires 'leadership' and 'followership'. In situations where PHA is delivered, it is common that multiagency teams may have never worked together before. The obstacles this can create must be quickly managed. When arriving on scene it is important to identify the key multiagency staff members (senior ambulance officer / fire officer etc.) to liaise with. Introductions and the early establishment of skill levels, knowledge and roles within the newly formed team, facilitate the efficient use of all team members. It is important that one person is identified as being in control at any given time, and this leader has the role of coordinating the activities of the team. When possible the leader should maintain an overview of the situation and task. For a Doctor this may mean a hands-off approach in relation to the patient for much of the task, with patient contact only for critical interventions that cannot be delegated.

The individual taking the leadership role may change dynamically throughout the different phases of the task, but in order to maintain just one leader at any given time, this role should be clearly handed over. An example of this may be the Fire Officer controlling the scene safety and access to the patient, then the doctor leading patient assessment to ascertain urgency of extrication, a second Fire Officer co-ordinating extrication, the Helicopter Emergency Medical Service (HEMS) doctor leading the PHA to successful completion, then the HEMS paramedic overseeing the packaging and transfer of the patient to the aircraft.

Managing the task involves: planning ahead, prioritising, communicating with the team, identifying and utilising resources and ensuring that standards are maintained. In briefing the team, the leader should share their mental model of the task, whilst being open to suggestions from all other team-members. This should create a 'flattened' hierarchy, despite existing ranks and status, where all members of the team feel able to contribute ideas and concerns.

It is important to be a leader that others want to follow, demonstrating polite respect for all team-members, inspiring confidence, using authority and graded assertiveness as required, and avoiding and managing any conflict within the group. A 'tactical talk through' is often useful in maintaining the shared mental model. By explaining thoughts and reasoning, other members of the team are able to understand the situation and respond more appropriately to the leader's requests. Where problems arise and clinical circumstances are deteriorating, acknowledging and sharing this early allows the team to react in good time e.g., "I can't see the vocal cords at all, I can only just see the tip of the epiglottis and there is a lot of blood in the airway", allows the other team members to anticipate the requirement for additional suction, and preparation of additional kit for a difficult/failed intubation.

4.4   Communication

Communication is essential within the pre-hospital team to create the shared understanding required and to drive tasks forward. Communication can be considered as three components: the message (i.e., the information that needs to be passed), the sender of the message and the receiver of the message.

When working in a time-pressured environment, messages need to be concise and clear in their wording. Information that is not immediately relevant should be omitted. A large part of communication takes place on non-verbal levels, in 'how' we say something, and body language conveyed. Volume, pitch and intonation of voice are also powerful tools.

It is important that the 'receiver' of the information is ready to receive. Asking 'someone' to undertake a task often results in nobody doing it. Direct eye contact or use of names works well. Physical contact, such as touching the shoulder or arm, also gains attention when required. For information that must be shared with all of the team, (e.g., a safety concern) loud, clear and specific words (i.e., 'Stop, listen in') may be used to create a pause in activity and gain everyone's attention.

The empowerment of all staff to speak up is essential for patient safety. Despite best intentions, the pre-hospital team can often still have a hierarchical feel to it, with the doctor at the top. CUS (Box 4.3) is an acronym derived from the United Airlines' safety programme (Leonard et al. 2004). It provides an accepted way for someone who may feel lower in the team hierarchy to get the attention of someone higher up if they feel that there is a critical safety situation. It is designed as a 3-step escalating process.

Box 4.3: CUS
- **C**   'I'm Concerned'
- **U**   'I'm Uncomfortable'
- **S**   'This is a Safety Issue'

Closing the loop of communication is also important. This ensures that information has been received, and the correct action has taken place. When critical information is passed in the pre-hospital environment, noise and a narrow bandwidth may act as barriers to communication. It is therefore useful to repeat back and confirm important information: "You want me to give 70, seven zero, mg of Rocuronium, that is 7 ml?" and "Rocuronium given".

Having a recognised system for handover facilitates effective communication. The ATMIST format (Box 4.4) is now used widely both pre-hospital and particularly in the Emergency Department. It acts as an aid to delivering a concise and relevant message, whilst ensuring important information is not missed:

Box 4.4: ATMIST Handover
Age
Time of incident
Mechanism
Injuries
Signs
Treatment given

4.5   Decision-Making

Decisions have to be based on the available information, which is often incomplete. Good decision-making is based on identifying options, and balancing risks and benefits. As circumstances change (e.g., a patient suddenly deteriorating), an earlier decision (e.g., careful extrication on a long-board) may need re-evaluating. Decision-making on scene should involve the input of doctors, paramedics and other agency staff, all of who bring differing experience and perspectives to the team.

In a time-pressured situation, it is important to avoid cognitive biases. Our previous experience and learning has a large influence on the decisions we make. We develop information processing shortcuts, known as heuristics, to allow decisions to be made. These 'rules of thumb' may serve us well, and aid rapid decision-making. They can, however, result in the incorrect decision when the first available information is accepted without actively seeking further clarification and detail. This can result in a decision influenced by a recent experience that is not truly representative of the current situation.

Confirmation biases can also occur. This is when we tend to ignore evidence that does not support our initial theory, and attribute greater value to information that does. An example of this would be attending a well-known local 'drunk' found lying in the street and wrongly attributing his altered Glasgow Coma Score (GCS) to intoxication. The previous history of admissions with reduced GCS due to excess alcohol, a strong smell of alcohol, unkempt appearance, and a half drunk bottle of cider beside him provide confirmation bias to your presumed diagnosis. You do not think too hard about a witness account stating he had only purchased the bottle of cider from a nearby off-licence only 45 mins earlier and that the ambulance paramedic thinks one pupil is slightly larger than the other. He had probably been drinking earlier and the cider is extra strong after all...the difference in pupil size is minimal and probably within normal variation... As a result you leave him to be transferred to the nearest hospital by ambulance rather than intubating him and flying him to a trauma centre with neurosurgery that is further away. He deteriorates further in the ambulance, and aspirates en route to hospital. A CT scan subsequently reveals a large subdural haematoma requiring transfer to the neurosurgery unit by road 2 hrs later.

Awareness of all the factors that may be influencing your decision should reduce decision-making errors.

4.6 Task Management

When 'task fixation' occurs, the most critical problem may be ignored. This can be seen during a failed intubation, where activity is focused on achieving intubation rather than maintaining oxygenation.

Errors are more likely to occur at times of high cognitive load. Checklists are frequently utilised to minimise the chance of omission or incorrect action, for example: Pre-take-off checklist, Pre-RSI Checklist (See Appendices). Such checklists allow cognitive offloading, as these steps do not require memory recall. They ensure that critical steps are always considered and not missed. Use of a two person, 'challenge and response' checklist is recommended.

Standard Operating Procedures (SOPs) also have a role in enabling rapid decision-making (Box 4.5). When working in an environment with endless variables and high risk of errors, standardisation of factors such as equipment and processes, can be addressed at organisational level through the development of SOPs. These detail the agreed way in which the organisation requires a procedure to be carried out, are evidence-based where possible, and are subject to regular review and updates. They serve to reduce variability in practice, supporting the delivery of safe and reproducible, high quality medical care. For example, there are a multitude of drug combinations that could theoretically be used to induce anaesthesia in a trauma patient. An SOP with one combination of drugs to use (perhaps with one or two exceptions) removes this clinical debate, and allows attentions to be focused on other decisions. SOPs also provide a standard for practice to be audited against.

Box 4.5: SOPs Commonly Utilised for PHA
- **Equipment** – equipment to be carried and packed in a certain way
- **Pre-Hospital RSI** – ensures a consistent and safe process whichever team members are working together
- **Drugs** – a limited selection of drugs carried and prepared at standard concentrations
- **Difficult/failed intubation** – an agreed protocol ensures rapid response to a critical event

4.7   Training

Training is an essential part of CRM, both in understanding the concepts and in rehearsing procedures. Analogous to flight simulation, moulage scenario training using manikin simulators allows challenging unfamiliar situations to be encountered in a safe environment.

A Pre-Hospital Anaesthesia course is an excellent place to start, however, regular training within individual organisations, even if this is only a 5 min run through of an SOP, is necessary to maintain a high level of performance.

Box 4.6
'Under pressure you don't rise to the occasion, you sink to the level of your training'
  US pilot and author Barrett Tillman

References

Cooper GE, White MD, Lauber JK. Resource management on the flightdeck: proceedings of a NASA/industry workshop. (NASA CP-2120). Moffett Field: NASA-Ames Research Center; 1980.

Endsley MR. Designing for situation awareness in complex systems. Proceedings of the Second international workshop on symbiosis of humans, artifacts and environment, Kyoto. 2001. http://www.researchgate.net/publication/238653506_Designing_for_situation_awareness_in_complex_system.

European Organisation for the Safety of Air Navigation. Guidelines for developing and implementing team resource management. 1996. https://www.eurocontrol.int/sites/default/files/content/documents/nm/safety/safety-guidelines-for-developing-and-implementing-team-resource-management-1996.pdf. Accessed 02 Jun 2015.

Federal Aviation Authority. http://www.faa.gov/regulations_policies/handbooks_manuals/aviation/risk_management_handbook/media/rmh_ch03.pdf. Accessed 05 Feb 2015.

Leonard M, Graham S, Bonacum D. The human factor: the critical importance of effective teamwork and communication in providing safe care. Qual Saf Health Care. 2004;13 Suppl 1:i85–90. doi:10.1136/qshc.2004.010033.

Reason J. Human error: models and management. BMJ. 2000; 320:768–70.

Chapter 5
Post-intubation Management

At the end of this chapter you should:

• Understand the importance of post-intubation care
• Know the ABCDEF approach to pre-transfer checks

The quality of care delivered after intubation and during transfer to hospital may have as much influence on outcome as the intubation itself. Experience from intrahospital transfers suggests that unexpected problems or complications occur in around 65 % of transfers, with critical or life-threatening incidents occurring in nearly 9 % (Lovell et al. 2001; Papson et al. 2007). In the pre-hospital environment the incidence of complications can be expected to be higher, as the environment is often less controlled and the patient more unstable. Lovell et al. commented that many of the difficulties were preventable with adequate pre-transport communication and planning.

Intubating a patient increases the burden of patient monitoring and complicates the transfer. The patient can no longer protect their own airway, they are unable to ventilate themselves effectively or communicate the potential for deterioration or further injury. Additional equipment is required to adequately monitor their vital signs and ventilation. Vigilance is essential to avoid accidental extubation, disconnection, and decannulation. It is possible to minimise these risks by careful packaging and meticulous monitoring during the transfer to

T. Lowes et al., *Pre-Hospital Anesthesia Handbook*, 99
DOI 10.1007/978-3-319-23090-0_5,
© Springer-Verlag London 2016

hospital. Minimum monitoring standards are essential for the safe transfer of intubated patients in the pre-hospital environment. Ventilators and monitors should include audible alarms which can be heard easily (through headsets if necessary), and visual alarms that can be seen clearly during transfer.

Long distance transfer of critically ill patients *can* be achieved without any major complications in the setting of a dedicated transfer team (Uusaro et al. 2002). It is reasonable to assume that a dedicated and well-trained pre-hospital team should also minimise, if not eliminate, the incidence of major complications on route to hospital. The transfer of intubated patients between hospitals is usually carried out by anaesthetists (Jameson and Lawler 2000), but a large number of pre-hospital intubations and subsequent transfers are not. For non-anaesthetists who are not used to transferring critically ill ventilated patients, there is a lot to remember. An ABCDEF approach (utilising a checklist) should make this easier. This system is also recommended for those who consider themselves experienced transfer doctors. The stress of managing a critically ill patient in a pre-hospital environment can easily result in incomplete preparation and an increased risk of adverse events.

Pre-transport planning and preparation in a structured manner is therefore the focus of this chapter. After intubation and before transfer a full check should be performed.

5.1   A (and C-Spine) BCDEF Approach

5.1.1   Airway (Box 5.1)

The airway only remains protected as long as the endotracheal tube (ETT) cuff remains inflated below the vocal cords. For this reason it must be secure. This can be achieved using either adhesive tape or a fabric tie. Both techniques have their limitations. Tape is unlikely to provide adequate security in the presence of rain, sweat, grease, blood, or facial hair. Fabric tube ties overcome these issues, however, if applied too tightly, can lead to venous congestion and increased intracranial pressure. For this reason, tape should be used preferentially for head-injured patients. This can be made even more secure by splitting the tape longitudinally (like trouser legs) and wrapping around the tube. Zinc oxide tape is preferred by many operators, as its gets more adhesive as it warms up. Alternatively others recommend more expensive proprietary fixation devices, which may hold the ETT more securely. The Thomas™ ETT holder allowed significantly less ETT displacement when compared to a tied tape in a manikin study (Murdoch and Holdgate 2007).

Flexion and extension of the head can lead to migration of the ETT. This is particularly relevant in children where smaller anatomy means that relatively small movements can result in either endobronchial intubation or extubation. Although in children, flexion appears to consistently cause downward displacement of the tube (distance relative to age) and extension causes upward movement, in adults the movement can be either way (up to 2 cm down or 3 cm out) (Weiss et al. 2006; Yap et al. 1994). In an adult the ETT cuff should be placed 2 cm below the cords to minimise the risk of problems occurring. Some ETTs are marked at the distal end to provide an indication of optimal positioning. The mark on the tube should usually be positioned just through the vocal cords.

In adults, the left main bronchus is narrower and branches off the trachea at more of an acute angle compared with the right; hence endobronchial intubation is invariably right-sided. The incidence of endobronchial intubation can be reduced by ensuring the presence of bilateral breath sounds and chest movement after securing the tube in position. Endobronchial intubation should be suspected in the presence of unexpectedly high airway pressures during ventilation. Bronchospasm may also be an indicator of endobronchial intubation or the potential for it (the bronchospasm may be due to carinal irritation). Withdrawing the ETT by 2 cm is usually adequate to improve the situation.

When the ETT is positioned satisfactorily, note the measurement at the teeth (usually 22–24 cm for an adult). This may then be used as a reference point if there are concerns that the tube has migrated during transfer. This information should be recorded and communicated on handover.

Prolonged ETT cuff inflation pressures of greater than 30 cm H_2O can lead to tracheal mucosa ischaemia (Seegobin and van Hasselt 1984). This is unlikely to be an issue during transport following pre-hospital anaesthesia (PHA) within the UK due to relatively short transfer times. If longer journey times are expected, consideration should be given to monitoring and adjusting pressures with a simple hand-held device. This is more relevant when travelling by air, when *actual* cuff pressure remains the same but *actual* mucosal capillary pressure is lower (although the same relative to atmospheric pressure). Alternatively the air can be exchanged for saline, although it can be difficult to adjust cuff pressure using this.

Effective suction must always accompany the intubated patient. Both Yankauer (oropharyngeal) and endobronchial catheters should be available for airway toileting en route. More recent tubes have suction ports above the cuff to allow for regular suction of oropharyngeal secretions, which tend to pool above the cuff in the unconscious patient. In the intensive care setting, subglottic suction ETTs have been shown to decrease the incidence of ventilator associated pneumonia (Muscedere et al. 2011). If a patient is being transferred to a unit using these, it is preferable to use this type of tube for PHA to avoid unnecessary tube change at a later stage.

A heat moisture exchange filter (HMEF) should always be used between the patient and the ventilator circuit. This protects the ventilator equipment from contamination and allows some moisture and heat exchange between the inspired and expired gases. Cold dry inspired gases can increase heat loss and degrade the function of respiratory cilia.

Box 5.1: Post-intubation Airway Check
- Secure tube
- Check position
- Suction available
- HMEF

5.1.2   Cervical Spine (Box 5.2)

One in every nine trauma patients requiring intubation will have a cervical spine injury. Of these, one third will be unstable (Patterson 2004). Therefore it is not unreasonable to assume that every severely injured trauma patient may have an unstable neck injury and treat them as such.

A long spinal board and a semi-rigid collar are often used for extrication of casualties in Road Traffic Collisions (RTCs). The spinal board may then be used for onward transfer to hospital. Prolonged periods of immobilisation on a spinal board can lead to the development of pressure necrosis. This is more likely to occur in the hypotensive patient because of reduced tissue perfusion. The skin overlying bony prominences in contact with the spinal board is most at risk (scapulae, sacrum, and heels). The long spinal board is also not a good spinal splint as it allows a significant degree of lateral movement. Therefore it should be considered only as an extrication device. Increasingly a scoop stretcher is used for pre-hospital transfer of trauma patients. It confers advantages of requiring less rolling and movement of the patient , and offers more stability against lateral spinal movement. If transfer times are likely to be prolonged (e.g., >30 min), the patient should be "scooped" onto a vacuum mattress and the spinal board used purely for supporting the mattress during transfer between vehicles/trolleys. When a patient is transferred on a long spinal board or a scoop stretcher, it should be removed as soon as possible on arrival in the Emergency Department (i.e., on completion of the primary survey) (Vickery 2001).

Semi-rigid collars are also associated with significant morbidity. Inappropriate sizing can lead to raised intracranial pressure (ICP). It is important to ensure that no clothing is trapped under the collar as this may result in skin injury and inadequate stabilisation. It is essential that correct sizing and fitting takes place on scene. These collars often remain in situ for a considerable time prior to definitive management, and some hospital staff may have limited experience in their use. Secure head blocks (or fluid/sand bags with tape) are also required to ensure full cervical spine immobilisation.

Box 5.2: Post-intubation Cervical Spine Check
- Collar sized and fitted correctly
- Consider vacuum mattress

5.1.3   Breathing (Box 5.3)

Manual ventilation cannot provide reliable and consistent minute ventilation (Cardman and Friedman 1997). It is also labour intensive and limits concurrent activity. Mechanical ventilators address both these issues. Even when mechanical ventilation is employed, optimal oxygenation and ventilation cannot be assured (Helm et al. 2003). End-tidal CO_2 ($ETCO_2$) must be used for any intubated ventilated patient, as it can be used to judge the adequacy of ventilation. The waveforms can also be useful for the recognition of trends in ventilation and diagnosing ventilatory problems (Fig. 5.1).

5.1.4   Over Ventilation or Fall in Cardiac Output

The normal $PaCO_2 - ETCO_2$ gradient is between 0.3 and 0.7 kPa (Bhavani-Shankar et al. 1992). Unfortunately $ETCO_2$ is only predictive of the trend in $PaCO_2$ in 77 % of ventilated patients. Hypovolaemic patients and patients with severe lung contusions are most likely to have a greater difference between $PaCO_2$ and $ETCO_2$ (pathological increase in dead space). These patients may have gradients as high as 1.5 kPa. The delivery of carbon dioxide to the lungs is dependent primarily on pulmonary blood flow. If ventilator settings

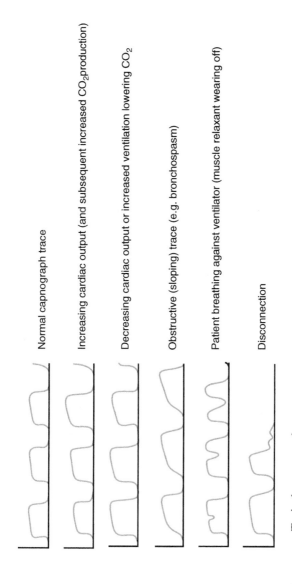

Normal capnograph trace

Increasing cardiac output (and subsequent increased CO_2 production)

Decreasing cardiac output or increased ventilation lowering CO_2

Obstructive (sloping) trace (e.g. bronchospasm)

Patient breathing against ventilator (muscle relaxant wearing off)

Disconnection

FIGURE 5.1 Typical capnograph traces

remain unchanged then an increase in $ETCO_2$ implies an improvement in total body cardiac output (Falk 1993). Similarly, a reduction in $ETCO_2$ should provoke a reassessment of the circulation before simply reducing the minute ventilation.

When using a mechanical ventilator, a self-inflating Bag-valve-mask (BVM) must always be taken as a backup. It not only allows ventilation in the event of mechanical failure but can also be used to hand ventilate via the face mask in the event of accidental extubation. To ensure adequate oxygenation in this situation, it is necessary to have a flow meter adapter on one of the oxygen cylinders and oxygen tubing (sized to fit the flow meter) attached to the bag. Modern lightweight cylinders will usually have both Schrader and "fir tree" connectors which makes things easier.

Before departure calculate the maximum oxygen requirement for the journey and confirm that sufficient is being carried (see under *ventilators* later). Make a note of the Peak airway pressure – if this changes during transfer, a problem is developing or has occurred (e.g., ETT moved into bronchus, tension pneumothorax, etc.).

Reassess the chest before starting the transfer. This is probably the last chance to auscultate the chest prior to arrival in hospital. The patient has been ventilated for a few minutes by this stage and if a tension pneumothorax is developing, it should be apparent by now. This allows appropriate management to take place prior to departure rather than during transfer.

Box 5.3: Post-intubation Breathing Check
- Mechanical ventilator settings and oxygen requirements
- BVM available
- Reassess the chest

5.1.5   Circulation (Box 5.4)

Intravenous (IV) access should be checked for patency and security prior to transfer. A cannula falling out during transfer may be at best inconvenient and at worst a disaster. Reestablishing venous access whilst on the move is invariably difficult. A cannula should be secured with tape rather than just a dressing. Most dressings do not provide direct counter-traction to the cannula being pulled out. They often simply lie over the top of the cannula, keeping the site clean. The cannula should be fixed so that it cannot be tugged out of the vein nor can it be lifted up from the skin and kinked over. In addition, the IV giving set tubing should be secured to the arm. Incorporating a loop provides additional protection.

The blood pressure should be monitored closely during transfer, either by regular automatic cycling (3–5 min) or, in ongoing haemorrhage, by palpation of the radial pulse.

Intubated trauma patients are a heterogeneous group. Age, physiological reserve, pattern and severity of injury, and individual response to injury all differ. Similarly: entrapment, current physiological status, proximity to definitive care, and mode of transport all influence fluid administration decisions. As discussed earlier; the optimal pre-hospital fluid resuscitation strategy is not clear. Patients that are bleeding acutely can be separated into two groups: controllable and uncontrollable haemorrhage.

The controllable haemorrhage group includes soft tissue trunk injury and extremity trauma. In this group, haemorrhage can be controlled at scene by direct pressure, pressure dressings, proximal arterial pressure, or tourniquet. Fluid should be administered to these patients if evidence of hypoperfusion is present. The aim of management should be to achieve a good volume radial pulse and the improvement of $ETCO_2$ but not achieving normovolaemia.

In the uncontrollable haemorrhage group, rapid transfer to definitive care is the key to survival. Fluid should be given if there is a marked reduction of $ETCO_2$, loss of radial pulse or systolic pressure falls below 80 mmHg. Otherwise, fluids should be connected and ready to run if required. A fluid bolus may also be considered if severe tachycardia or signs of heart strain are evident on the electrocardiograph (ECG).

Tranexamic acid (TXA) is an antifibrinolytic that competitively inhibits the activation of Plasminogen to Plasmin. Plasmin is responsible for breaking down fibrin in blood clots. TXA therefore prevents the excessive breakdown of blood clots that can occur as part of the acute coagulopathy of trauma (ACoT) (Brohi et al. 2007). It can therefore reduce ongoing blood loss in haemorrhagic shock. TXA (15 mg/kg) should be routinely given to all patients with (or at risk of) significant haemorrhage (i.e., enough to cause peripheral vasoconstriction and tachycardia). This is supported by the CRASH-2 trial (CRASH-2 2010).

Burns casualties and patients with crush injuries (providing they do not also have uncontrollable haemorrhage) should be managed to achieve normal cardiovascular parameters, and will need significant amounts of fluid within the first 24 h post-injury. This should ideally be a balanced crystalloid, to prevent hyperchloraemic acidosis resulting from repeated infusion of 0.9 % NaCl. Fluid resuscitation and the management of hypotension is also discussed in Chap. 3.

An ECG may be susceptible to interference during transfer; however it is part of minimum monitoring. If the pulse oximeter is not reading, the ECG will be providing the only visual representation of heart rate. ST segment changes may suggest hypoxia, reduced cardiac output, or an acute coronary syndrome. The ECG may also indicate that the cause of sudden hypotension is a dysrhythmia rather than hypovolaemia. This may require treatment with cardioversion, rather than persisting blindly (and inappropriately) with fluid therapy.

It is also important to note that pelvic injuries are commonly underdiagnosed. These injuries can lead to catastrophic bleeding during transfer yet can be very difficult to detect in the pre-hospital environment. "Springing" the pelvis is very insensitive and may cause marked hypotension if an unstable fracture is present, so cannot be advocated. In any trauma patient, when pelvic injury cannot be excluded, a binder or pelvic sling should be applied as early as possible. Similarly, limb fractures should be splinted for transfer to minimise further blood loss (and pain).

> **Box 5.4: Post-intubation Circulation Check**
> - Haemorrhage control
> - Secure IV access
> - Monitor BP/pulse/ECG
> - Fluids vs. no fluids
> - TXA

5.1.6   Disability (Box 5.5)

The safe transfer of an intubated patient requires adequate muscle relaxation for the duration of the transfer. If Rocuronium 1.2 mg/kg is used for pre-hospital rapid sequence intubation (PRSI), this will normally maintain neuromuscular blockade for up to an hour. If Suxamethonium was used, a non-depolarising muscle relaxant (e.g., Rocuronium or Vecuronium) should be given prior to transfer. Muscle relaxation will ensure absolute immobility and ventilator synchrony during transfer, and this enhances patient stability. The main risk of paralysis for the patient is awareness. Being conscious, yet paralysed and unable to communicate pain and discomfort (from either trauma or intubation) can be a very distressing experience. To prevent this, the use of paralysis also mandates the use of adequate sedation. Patients who have a low Glasgow Coma Score (GCS) prior to intubation should also be provided with some form of sedation for two reasons: firstly, improvements in oxygenation and cardiac output secondary to medical intervention may well result in improved cerebral oxygenation and subsequent improvement in the level of consciousness. Secondly, these patients will still mount a sympathetic response to the presence of an ETT in the trachea or to the manipulation of injuries during handling. These sympathetic responses may aggravate raised intracranial pressure or lead to myocardial ischaemia.

Always check and document pupil response again prior to transfer; there may have been a change following intubation and ventilation. Adequate anaesthesia should result in central and equal pupils that still show some response to light (this is not affected by neuromuscular blockade). Opioids will cause miosis, but the sympathomimetic effect of Ketamine may negate this effect.

The presence of unilateral pupillary dilatation should be assumed to be a sign of raised intracranial pressure until proven otherwise (it may possibly be due to direct trauma or previous surgery). The appearance of pupillary dilatation after initial normal appearance is indicative of an expanding intracranial haematoma. Urgent transfer to a neurosurgical centre for evacuation of haematoma is crucial. Mannitol (0.25–0.5 g/kg) or hypertonic saline (e.g., 2 mls/kg of 5 % NaCl) should be given and temporary mild hyperventilation may be considered appropriate.

As the patient is now sedated and paralysed, they will no longer be able to protect their own eyes. Monitoring leads, fluid tubing, and blankets are all liable to be dragged across a patient's face and may cause corneal abrasion unless the eyes are covered (e.g., taped closed). External elements of wind, dust and debris are also an issue. Tape can be lifted to allow ongoing assessment of pupillary size and reactivity during transfer.

Box 5.5: Post-intubation Disability Check
- Paralysis AND sedation
- Protect eyes but monitor pupils

5.1.7   Exposure and Packaging (Box 5.6)

Performing a full secondary survey following PRSI is not appropriate. Any potential sources of bleeding (including long bone, abdominal, and pelvic injury) should have been identified. Ensure that no major injuries to the patient's back have been missed (particularly wounds which may indicate intrathoracic or intraabdominal injury). In most cases, hypothermia should now be avoided. Anaesthesia will cause peripheral vasodilation and loss of autoregulation of body temperature, causing the patient to cool down unless appropriate measures are taken. The patient should be covered with blankets to both reflect heat and to deflect rain and wind. These must be secure, particularly if transfer is by helicopter when loose articles become a serious hazard.

During the transfer of a sedated and paralysed patient it is the responsibility of the medical attendant to prevent further injury. This includes ensuring that the patient is securely strapped to the stretcher/spinal board prior to a move. Limbs are particularly at risk whilst carrying and fitting stretchers into ambulances and aircraft. They should also be sufficiently padded to prevent pressure necrosis or direct nerve injury (e.g., ulna nerve at the elbow), prior to longer transfers.

It is important to leave access to IV lines in case drugs need to be given urgently during transfer. Leaving the hand and wrist uncovered also permits easy assessment of the radial pulse.

Patients with head-injuries should ideally be nursed with a 15° head-up tilt. This improves venous drainage and reduces ICP.

Box 5.6: Post-intubation Exposure Check
- Assess for potential source of blood loss and injuries to the back
- Prevent exposure (allowing IV access)

5.1.8   (F)Phone Ahead

Finally, before transferring the patient to hospital, a member of the team should phone the receiving hospital to warn them of your imminent arrival. This is particularly important when a full trauma team (including urgent radiology), or specialist service (e.g., Cardiology Percutaneous Coronary Intervention (PCI)) is likely to be required. This allows time to ensure all relevant staff are present and prepared for the arrival of your patient.

5.1.9   Handover and Documentation

Despite the urgency of the situation; clear, comprehensive and contemporaneous records must be kept. This is usually in the format of a Patient Record Form (PRF) (Fig 5.2). This includes: patient details, injuries found, monitored observations, interventions performed and drugs given, along with timings.

It is important to communicate effectively with the receiving team members and ensure that the tempo of resuscitation and management is not lost. The initial verbal handover is best delivered in the form of ATMIST (Box 5.7). Other specific and relevant information can then be added (e.g., Allergies and significant Past Medical History). An indication of the progress of the patient while in your care will give valuable information about the requirement for further investigation or intervention (e.g., 'They have been stable throughout transfer' vs SpO_2 has been falling during transfer'). Any critical events or difficulties (e.g., with intubation) should also be reported.

Box 5.7: ATMIST Handover
- **A**ge of patient
- **T**ime of Injury
- **M**echanism
- **I**njuries
- **S**igns and symptoms
- **T**reatment

Ideally a full AMPLE history (Box 5.8) along with the name of the patient and next of kin information should then be handed over to hospital staff along with a copy of the pre-hospital PRF. A ventilated patient must only be handed over to an individual capable of caring for them, i.e., an experienced anaesthetist in most cases. If not immediately

COMPLETE EVERY SECTION OR CROSS OUT BOX							
GNAAS PATIENT REPORT FORM	Location		Mobile	On scene		PRF No.	
	Medic 1		AT PT			Date	
			Left Scene			Heli	
Airbase Tel:	Medic 2		Hospital			Car Amb	

Incident Description & Time		Weight	Patient Name & Address				
		kg	D.O.B				

Injury Description & Management	Time					
	ECG					
	Pulse					
	B/P					
	R.R.					
	Pain Score 1-10					
	Spo_2					
	GCS E					
	V					
	M					
	$ETCO_2$					
	DRUGS	Time/Dose		Time/Dose		Time/Dose
	Fentanyl					
	Ketamine					
	Rocuronium					
	Morphine					
	Midazolam					
	Tranexamic Acid					

A	PATIENT CONSENT	Limb MVT	O/S	Reason	
B	Informed ☐	RA	Y/N	Time	
				Soiling	
C	Presumed ☐	RL	Y/N	Length	
		LA	Y/N	C&L Grade	
D AVPU	Refused ☐ Please sign appropriate	LL	Y/N	Tube Size	
Handover / Comments	Medic 1			Pupil Size L R	pre RSI
	Medic 2			Blankets	Y / N
	Handover			Self Discharge	Capacity Y / N
Hospital Triage MHP ☐	Time				

Figure 5.2 Patient Report Form (PRF)

available, the pre-hospital clinician should be prepared to remain with the patient for a short time until a suitable doctor is available for handover.

Box 5.8: The AMPLE History
- **A**llergies
- **M**edications
- **P**ast Medical History
- **L**ast meal
- **E**vents leading to injury

After handover is complete, the team should clean their equipment and replenish their consumables so they are ready for further tasking. A duplicate full set of prepacked equipment may facilitate a rapid turnaround.

5.2   Conclusion

Successful PRSI is only the start of the journey. The management of the ventilated critically ill patient during transfer to hospital is just as important as the interventions on scene. The post-intubation period is an opportunity to continue resuscitation; however, it also has the potential to increase morbidity and mortality. Using a simple ABCDEF system prior to transfer can reduce the chance of adverse events and ensure optimum management should unexpected problems occur.

References

Bhavani-Shankar K, Moseley H, Kumar AY, Delph Y. End-tidal carbon dioxide. Can J Anaesth. 1992;39:617–32.

Brohi K, Cohen MJ, Davenport RA. Acute coagulopathy of trauma: mechanism, identification and effect. Curr Opin Crit Care. 2007;13:680–5.

Cardman E, Friedman D. Further studies of manually operated self-inflating resuscitation bags. Anesth Anal. 1997;56:202–6.

CRASH-2 trial collaborators. Effects of tranexamic acid on death, vascular occlusive events, and blood transfusion in trauma. Lancet. 2010;376:23–32.

Falk JL. End-tidal carbon dioxide monitoring during cardiopulmonary resuscitation. Advances in anaesthesia. St. Louis: Mosby-Yearbook; 1993. p. 275–88.

Helm M, Schuster R, Hauke J, Lampl L. Tight control of pre-hospital ventilation by capnography in major trauma victims. Br J Anaesth. 2003;90:327–32.

Jameson PPM, Lawler PG. Transfer of critically ill patients in the northern region. Anaesthesia. 2000;55:489.

Lovell MA, Mudaliar MY, Klineberg PL. Intrahospital transport of critically ill patients: complications and difficulties. Anaesth Intensive Care. 2001;29:400–5.

Murdoch E, Holdgate A. A comparison of tape tying versus a tube-holding device for securing ETTs in adults. Anaesth Intensive Care. 2007;35:730–5.

Muscedere J, Rewa O, McKechnie K, et al. Subglottic secretion drainage for the prevention of ventilator-associated pneumonia: a systematic review and meta-analysis. Crit Care Med. 2011;39:1985–91.

Papson JP, Russell KL, Taylor DM. Unexpected events during the intrahospital transport of critically ill patients. Acad Emerg Med. 2007;14:574–7.

Patterson H. Emergency department intubation of trauma patients with undiagnosed spinal injury. Emerg Med J. 2004;21:302–5.

Seegobin RD, van Hasselt GL. Endotracheal cuff pressure and tracheal mucosal blood flow: endoscopic study of effects of four large volume cuffs. Br Med J (Clin Res Ed). 1984;288:965–8.

Uusaro A, Parviainen I, Takala J, Ruokonen E. Safe long-distance interhospital ground transfer of critically ill patients with acute severe unstable respiratory and circulatory failure. Intensive Care Med. 2002;28:1122–5.

Vickery D. The use of the spinal board after the pre-hospital phase of trauma management. Emerg Med J. 2001;18:51–4.

Weiss M, et al. Tracheal tube-tip displacement in children during headneck movement-a radiological assessment. Br J Anaesth. 2006;96:486–91.

Yap SJ, Morris RW, Pybus DA. Alterations in ETT position during general anaesthesia. Anaesth Intensive Care. 1994;22:586–8.

Chapter 6
Equipment and Minimum Monitoring Standards

By the end of this chapter you should know:

- What constitutes minimum monitoring standards.
- The equipment required to safely carry out pre-hospital anaesthesia (PHA).
- How to set a ventilator.
- How to perform an oxygen requirement calculation.

6.1 Monitoring

As with all forms of anaesthesia the most important monitor of patient well-being is the close attention of the clinician delivering it. Simple, but essential clinical measurement and monitoring should include:

- Pulse, rate and character (weak or strong); this may include distal pulses
- Respiratory rate
- Pupil size and reactivity
- Presence or absence of muscular activity and limb movement

In addition to this, electro-medical monitors markedly improve the safety of anaesthesia, especially in austere and confined environments. For this reason the minimum

T. Lowes et al., *Pre-Hospital Anesthesia Handbook*,
DOI 10.1007/978-3-319-23090-0_6,
© Springer-Verlag London 2016

monitoring standard to undertake PHA and onward patient transfer must be the same as in-hospital anaesthesia, and this is outlined in the Association of Anaesthetists and the Intensive Care Society safety guidance on Pre-hospital Anaesthesia (2000, 2009) (Whiteley et al. 2002) (Box 6.1).

Box 6.1: Minimum Monitoring Standards (Fig. 6.1)
- Pulse oximetry
- Continuous ECG monitoring
- Non-invasive blood pressure (NIBP)
- End-Tidal Carbon dioxide ($ETCO_2$) measurement

Exceptionally it may be necessary to reduce this level of monitoring during the extrication of trapped patients, but full monitoring must be re-established at the earliest opportunity. A small battery powered pulse oximeter that clips onto a

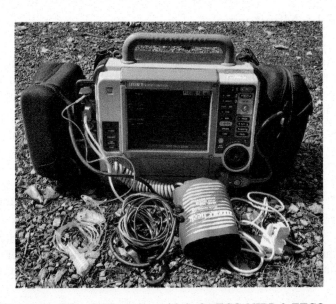

FIGURE 6.1 Lifepak 15 monitor with SpO_2, ECG, NIBP & $ETCO_2$

finger will at least provide heart rate and pulse oximetry. The absence of monitoring equipment is a strong contra-indication to pre-hospital anaesthesia. In the case of equipment failure a risk-benefit analysis should be undertaken to determine whether anaesthesia is still appropriate and the decision clearly written in the patient's notes.

NIBP measurements should be taken at least every 3 min during and following pre-hospital anaesthesia. It is important to be aware that frequent NIBP cycling may be a significant drain on a monitor battery. Batteries should be conditioned and maintained as per the manufacturers instructions and at least one spare should always be carried. Invasive arterial pressure monitoring uses far less energy, however this is impractical in most circumstances due to the additional time required to perform and set-up.

In addition to manual documentation of monitoring measurements, most monitors should now provide the ability to record, review and either download or print readings for future reference.

6.1.1 Capnography

$ETCO_2$ measurement *must* be quantitative (i.e. provide an accurate numeric value). A capnograph is the gold standard, as this provides a reassuring visual display of each breath and can be an additional sign of ventilator disconnection. Lightweight, battery powered, portable monitors are commercially available (e.g. Capnocheck® (Fig. 6.2)), although most pre-hospital defibrillator monitors now include waveform capnography as one of their functions. They use infrared absorbance spectroscopy to determine the presence and quantity of CO_2 in the exhaled breath. Monitors generally display this information as a figure and as a waveform. The waveforms can be useful for the recognition of trends in ventilation and diagnosing ventilatory problems. The shape of the trace can indicate problems such as a patient starting to breathe against the ventilator, or obstructive breathing (kinked tubing or bronchospasm (Fig. 5.1)). Some devices may need regular calibration.

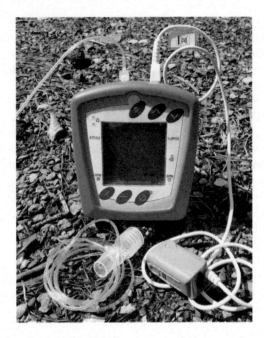

FIGURE 6.2 Capnocheck II battery powered capnograph

6.1.2   Capnometer

A capnometer (e.g. EMMA™ (Fig. 6.3)) is the next best
option. This will give an accurate figure to guide ventilation,
but no waveform. The final option is a qualitative $ETCO_2$
device. These only provide evidence of the presence of CO_2
and usually an idea of whether this is high or low, typically by
colour change (e.g. Easy Cap®(Figs. 6.4 and 6.5)). They are
disposable and consist of a filter paper impregnated with a
pH-sensitive, non-toxic chemical indicator that reversibly
changes colour on contact with CO_2. The Easy Cap® provides a breath to breath colour change from purple on inspiration to yellow on expiration, confirming the presence of
CO_2 in the exhaled breath. Qualitative devices are only really
suitable for confirmation of tracheal placement of a tube in
the absence or failure of a quantitative device, and should be
replaced as soon as possible.

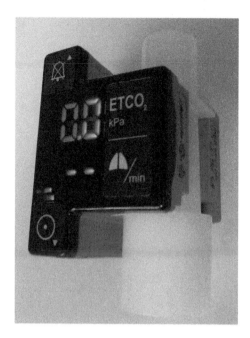

FIGURE 6.3 EMMA™ capnometer

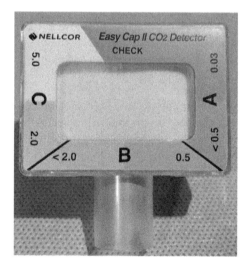

FIGURE 6.4 Easy Cap II – CO_2 present

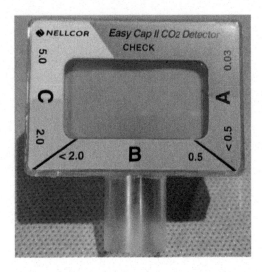

FIGURE 6.5 Easy Cap II – CO_2 absent

6.2   Other Equipment

All equipment used in the pre-hospital setting must be fit for purpose. It should be designed to allow it to be clinically effective, whilst meeting the demands of the operator. Of particular importance in pre-hospital use, it must be portable, robust and functional in a range of weather and environmental conditions. Visualisation of monitor screens must be possible from bright sunlight to darkness, and controls need to be both intuitive and easy to operate. Measurements should not be disturbed by vibration during transport; this is particularly relevant when travelling by helicopter. Alarm functions should involve multimodal alerting (e.g. noise *and* flashing lights) to overcome high ambient noise levels during transfer and bright light on scene. It should be noted that too many 'nuisance' alarms may distract from critical problems, and alarm limits may need amending to prevent this.

Battery life should be sufficient to comfortably provide time on scene, and onward transfer to hospital. Battery charging should follow the manufacturers guidance to ensure optimal performance, but back up batteries should always be carried.

To maintain an acceptable level of sterility, it is likely that much equipment will be disposable, similar to current day in-hospital practice.

Box 6.2 includes those items that are specifically required when performing PHA.

Box 6.2: Essential Equipment for Pre-Hospital RSI
- Laryngoscope handle and two laryngoscope blades (functioning light/batteries)
- Endotracheal tubes of appropriate size and length (lubricated) (Box 6.3)
- Suction apparatus with yankauer and flexible catheters
- Magill's forceps
- Bougie (Endotracheal tube introducer – *not* a stylet)
- 10 ml syringe for inflating the cuff
- Stethoscope
- Tape or tie to secure the endotracheal tube
- Catheter mount
- Heat Moisture Exchange Filter (HMEF)
- Capnograph or Capnometer
- Apparatus to ventilate the lungs (BVM *and* mechanical ventilator)

Equipment should also be immediately available for the management of difficult or failed intubation (Box 6.4).

Box 6.3: Suggested Sizes and Lengths for Endotracheal Tubes

Sizes: Male 8.0–9.0, Female 7.0–8.0, Children size = Age/4 + 4 cm (neonate 3.0)

Length to teeth: Male 22–24 cm, Female 20–22 cm, Children over 2 years Age/2 + 12 cm

Note: (1) Only open and cut tubes immediately prior to use (do not cut tubes in airway burns, anaphylaxis or trauma). (2) The cuff must always be tested prior to use.

Box 6.4: Equipment for Difficult or Failed Intubation

- Supraglottic airway (e.g. i-gel® (Fig. A.4) or LMA Proseal™(Fig. A.3))
- Emergency cricothyroidotomy kit (see Appendix E)
- Alternative laryngoscope (eg. McCoy Laryngoscope (Fig. 6.6), Airtraq™(Fig. 6.7), Glidescope® (Fig. 6.8) etc.)

All items of equipment should be checked daily against a list and where appropriate, correct functioning assured.

6.3   Ventilators

Transport ventilators range from the very simple to the complex and expensive versions that are essentially portable Intensive Care Unit (ICU) ventilators. The simplest ventilators are those that are gas driven and require no electrical supply to function. These are probably still the commonest

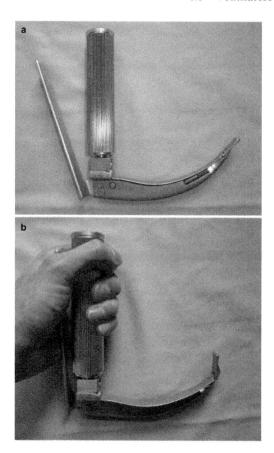

FIGURE 6.6 McCoy Laryngoscope (**a**). Initial 'resting' position for insertion of blade into vallecula. (**b**). Tip flexed by closing lever to lift epiglottis

found in use in the UK (e.g., Oxylog® 1000 (Fig. 6.9), ParaPAC™(Fig. 6.10) Moving up from these are ventilators which are still gas driven but allow the Inspiratory:Expiratory (I:E) ratios to be adjusted and provide a digital readout of ventilatory parameters e.g. Minute volume (e.g. Oxylog® 2000/3000).

Gas driven portable ventilators consume oxygen at a rate in excess of the set minute ventilation. This varies from 0.1 to

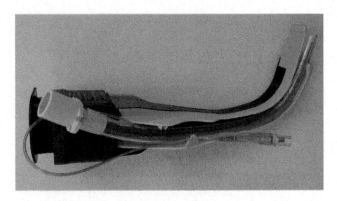

FIGURE 6.7 Airtraq™

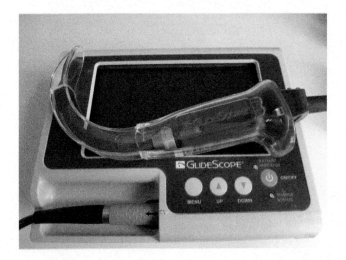

FIGURE 6.8 Glidescope™

1 L/min depending on the ventilator. Battery-powered ventilators have an internal turbine that draws in air from the
atmosphere and allows ventilation without a high-pressure
oxygen supply (although a cylinder is invariably connected to
provide the oxygen). These will therefore still function even if
the cylinder is empty but only provide a FiO$_2$ of 0.21 (Air). It
is essential for transferring personnel to be aware of the

7. Attach to patient and
note the generated
peak airway pressure

4. Set max pressure
alarm

3. No Air Mix = 100 % O_2
(Air Mix = 45–60 % O_2
depending on ventilator)

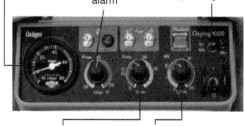

2. Set ventilation rate
(initially10/min in adults)
Aim for ETCO$_2$ 5.0kPa
(4–4.5kPa for head injury)

1. Set tidal volume (8mls/kg)

5. If available set Positive End Expiratory Pressure (PEEP)
on Ventilator or external valve (usual level = 5–15cm H_2O)

6. If available set I:E ratio. 1:1.5 ideal for ventilation,
1:2 or greater if hypovolaemic

FIGURE 6.9 Oxylog® 1000 ventilator

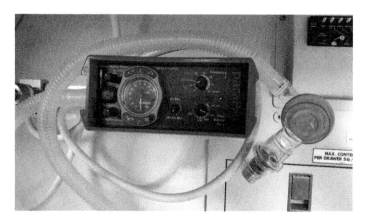

FIGURE 6.10 ParaPAC™ ventilator with external PEEP valve

technical specifications of the ventilator in use (including battery life and oxygen use) and account for these during planning. This data is available from the user manuals. Box 6.5 describes the minimum acceptable standard for a portable ventilator.

Box 6.5: Minimum Standard for a Portable Mechanical Ventilator
- Disconnection and high pressure alarms
- Ability to supply Positive End Expiratory Pressure
- Ability to vary the inspired oxygen concentration
- The ability to adjust the Inspiratory: Expiratory ratio, Respiratory Rate and Tidal Volume.

The oxygen requirement for the duration of the transfer should be calculated prior to departure (Box 6.6) and sufficient cylinders carried (Box 6.7). If logistics permit, twice the calculated volume of gas should accompany the patient to allow for unexpected delay. If this is not possible, a 60 mins reserve is the minimum acceptable.

Most ventilators possess a schraeder connector. Lightweight cylinders (e.g. CD size) have integral schraeder and fir tree connectors. Older cylinders must have a regulator attachment fitted. D and E size use a pin index regulator but the F size requires a bull nose connector. Different regulators and schraeder attachments may therefore need to be carried to ensure all cylinders are useable.

Box 6.6: How to Perform an Oxygen Requirement Calculation

Oxygen requirement = Ventilator dial setting (L / min)
$$+ \text{Ventilator driving gas requirement} (L / min)$$
$$\times \text{Journey time} (mins)$$

Ideally double the volume should be available

Box 6.7: Oxygen Cylinder Contents
D = 340 L
CD = 460 L
E = 680 L
F = 1360 L
ZX = 3040 L

Newer lightweight cylinders (i.e. CD, ZX) are ideal as they carry significantly more oxygen in a smaller and lighter container than steel cylinders.

6.3.1   How to Set a Ventilator (Fig. 6.9)

Ventilating patients with large tidal volumes (10–15 ml/kg) may lead to the release of inflammatory mediators (Slutsky and Tremblay 1998) and worsen Multiple Organ Dysfunction Syndrome (MODS) (Trembly et al. 1997). The adoption of a lung protective strategy in the intensive care unit appears to reduce mortality (The Acute Respiratory Distress Syndrome Network 2000). Critically ill patients intubated in the field are at risk of developing acute lung injury and MODS. For this reason, tidal volumes of 6–8 ml/kg body weight should be used. Peak airway pressures should be kept below 30 cmH$_2$O. If compliance is poor (airway pressures high relative to the tidal volume) the tidal volume should be reduced by 1 ml/kg to achieve this airway pressure. The ventilation rate should be set between 6 and 30/min to achieve an ETCO$_2$ below 5.5 kPa. Usually a rate of 10–12/min is appropriate. For patients with head injury, the aim should be to achieve an ETCO$_2$ of 4–4.5 kPa.

Increasing minute volume will tend to reduce venous return, particularly in hypovolaemic patients. This may lead to a marked decrease in cardiac output. Animal studies suggest that achieving adequate oxygenation with the lowest possible minute volume will result in better cardiac output and blood pressure (Pepe et al. 2003); therefore, start with a rate of 6–8 in hypovolaemic patients. $ETCO_2$ in these patients should not be a concern.

In head injured patients with hypovolaemia a compromise may have to be made. Either: give additional fluid to maintain blood pressure whilst ventilating to a normal $ETCO_2$ and accept the risk of further bleeding, or, hypoventilate (e.g., six breaths per min) to allow improved hemodynamics and potentially better brain oxygenation (whilst closely monitoring pupil reaction for signs of increasing intracranial pressure (ICP) subsequent to the increased $PaCO_2$) (Manley et al. 2000).

Positive end expiratory pressure (PEEP) can improve oxygenation and will minimise atelectasis in an anaesthetised patient. It should be routine to apply a PEEP of 5 cmH_2O to all patients and higher than this where there is evidence of lung contusion/collapse/consolidation/oedema, in order to improve oxygenation. PEEP has previously not been used routinely in patients with head injury; however, there is rarely any effect on ICP until PEEP is increased above 10 cmH_2O. As patients who have sustained a head injury or intracranial haemorrhage may often have aspirated prior to intubation, PEEP should be set just as it would be for other patients with consideration for risk/benefit if increasing above 10 cmH_2O.

PEEP may potentially exacerbate a reduction in blood pressure in those patients who are significantly hypovolaemic. The higher peak inspiratory pressure required to generate the same tidal volume results in a higher intrathoracic pressure, reduced venous return, and lower cardiac output. However if SpO_2 is persistently low despite 100 % oxygen the application of PEEP may still be required. Reducing the respiratory rate, as described earlier can minimise the effect on cardiac output.

The risk of tension pneumothorax increases with the onset of mechanical ventilation. Marked deterioration following intubation and ventilation should be managed according to the desaturation protocol (Appendix: Actions on Desaturation). If a tension pneumothorax is diagnosed it should be decompressed initially by needle thoracocentesis (Appendix: Needle Thoracocentesis). Progression to a formal definitive decompression with either a tube (Schmidt et al. 1998) or open thoracostomy (Appendix: Thoracostomy) (Deakin et al. 1995) depends on the patient's response and the proximity to definitive care. Prophylactic chest drain insertion is not recommended as it is not a benign procedure and may result in both immediate and delayed complications.

The severe asthmatic patient can be very difficult to ventilate, and every effort should be made to get them to hospital without inducing anaesthesia. If this is not possible, do not apply PEEP, reduce ventilation rate and set I:E at 1:3 to allow time for expiration.

Hyperoxaemia (excessive oxygen in the blood) may be considered harmful in the critically ill population, but it is inappropriate to limit oxygen administration in the pre-hospital setting, and the same applies to ventilating patients with chronic obstructive pulmonary disease (COPD); avoidance of hypoxia is the priority. It may, however, be necessary to use lower concentrations of oxygen (e.g., "Air-mix") if supplies are limited. In this situation the aim is to keep SpO_2 above 93 %. This equates to a PaO_2 of about 10 kPa in the majority of patients. The delivery of inspired oxygen concentration by portable ventilators may be completely variable or fixed (air-mix/no-air mix setting). The air-mix setting can equate to a FiO_2 of 0.45 or 0.6 depending on the ventilator.

References

AAGBI Safety Guideline. Pre-hospital anaesthesia. London: AAGBI; 2000.

Association of Anaesthetists of Great Britain and Ireland. Safety guideline: interhospital transfer. London: Association of Anaesthetists of Great Britain and Ireland; 2009.

Deakin CD, Davies G, Wilson A. Simple thoracostomy avoids chest drain insertion in pre-hospital trauma. J Trauma. 1995;39:373–4.

Manley GT, et al. Cerebral oxygenation during hemorrhagic shock: perils of hyperventilation and the therapeutic potential of hypoventilation. J Trauma. 2000;48:1025–32.

Pepe PE, et al. Emergency ventilatory management in hemorrhagic states: elemental or detrimental? J Trauma. 2003;54:1048–57.

Schmidt U, Salgo M, Gericii T, Blauch M, Maull KI, Tscherne H. Chest tube decompression of blunt chest injuries by physicians in the field: effectiveness and complications. J Trauma. 1998;44:98–101.

Slutsky AS, Tremblay LN. Multiple system organ failure: is mechanical ventilation a contributing factor? Am J Respir Crit Care Med. 1998;157:1751–5.

The Acute Respiratory Distress Syndrome Network. Ventilation with lower tidal volumes compared with traditional tidal volumes in acute lung injury and the acute respiratory distress syndrome. N Engl J Med. 2000;342:1301–8.

Trembly L, Valenza F, Ribeiro SP, Li J, Slutsky AS. Injurious strategies increase cytokines and c-fos m-RNA expression in an isolated rat lung model. J Clin Invest. 1997;99:944–52.

Whiteley S, Gray A, McHugh P, Riordan O'. Transport of the critically ill adult. London: Intensive Care Society Standards; 2002.

Chapter 7
Drugs and Sedation

By the end of this chapter you should:

- Know the dilution, dosing and indications of the drugs routinely used within PHA
- Appreciate the main side effects of these agents
- Understand the aim of sedation and sedation end points

The safety of pre-hospital anaesthesia (PHA) is very dependent on the familiarity of personnel with the techniques and drugs that they are using. Therefore, it is usual for well-developed pre-hospital systems to use a consistent technique and a limited number of drugs. All individuals involved with the drawing up and administration of these drugs should have an understanding of their pharmacology and pharmacokinetics.

The 'ideal' recipe for pre-hospital rapid sequence intubation (PRSI) is yet to be determined. Lyon et al. (2015) report the use of Fentanyl (3 mcg/kg), Ketamine (2 mg/kg) and Rocuronium (1 mg/kg) for the PRSI of trauma patients. This combination produced good conditions for laryngoscopy within 60 s, whilst maintaining favourable physiological parameters. The doses were reduced to Fentanyl 1 mcg/kg and Ketamine 1 mg/kg in those with haemodynamic compromise.

GNAAS advocates doses of 1–2 mcg/kg Fentanyl, 1–2 mg/kg Ketamine and 1.2 mg/kg Rocuronium (with the lower dose, or omission, of Fentanyl and lower dose of Ketamine in

T. Lowes et al., *Pre-Hospital Anesthesia Handbook*,
DOI 10.1007/978-3-319-23090-0_7,
© Springer-Verlag London 2016

hypotensive patients). A dose of 3 mcg/kg of Fentanyl is used in hypertensive patients with an isolated head injury.

7.1   Pre-treatment

Various drugs can be used to reduce the unwanted sympathetic response to laryngoscopy (hypertension, raised intracranial pressure (ICP)). Fentanyl 2 mcg/kg is a reasonable first choice, but should be used with caution in patients with cardiovascular instability, hypovolaemia or a systolic blood pressure (SBP) <120 mmHg. It has a peak effect at around 3 min, so would ideally be given 3 min prior to laryngoscopy. Unfortunately, it can cause respiratory depression and so there is potential for a period of hypoventilation between administration and induction if given early. To avoid this problem, whilst still obtunding the pressor response to laryngoscopy, it is possible to give Fentanyl in a higher dose (e.g. 3 mcg/kg) immediately prior to the induction agent. This allows a rapid induction whilst providing a similar effect to a lower dose even though the drug has not yet reached its peak effect. This risks delayed hypotension after the stimulation of laryngoscopy has receded. Lyon et al. (2015) reported the successful use of this higher dose, however they did note a higher number of patients with a 20 % reduction in blood pressure and hence advocated a reduced dose of 1 mcg/kg in patients with haemodynamic compromise.

Alfentanil has a peak effect within approximately 90 s and as such is theoretically a better choice than Fentanyl, however it is more prone to causing bradycardia and, more importantly, most clinicians are less familiar with Alfentanil and there is much less evidence of its use in RSI compared to Fentanyl. As Fentanyl is also useful as an analgesic in pre-hospital medicine, it seems sensible to only carry one potent opioid to cover both induction and analgesia.

There is little evidence of benefit from the use of Lidocaine to prevent an increase in ICP during RSI (Butler and Jackson 2002) and none in the pre-hospital environment, nor in comparison to Fentanyl. Lidocaine is therefore not recommended.

7.1.1   Fentanyl

This is a synthetic opioid. It is approximately 100 times more potent than Morphine.

Indication	Attenuate response to laryngoscopy e.g. in isolated head injury
	Rapid acting (but relatively short-lived) analgesia
Presentation	Clear solution containing 50 mcg/mL (2 mL amp)
Dilution for use	Neat
Dose	1–2 mcg/kg IV for analgesia, 1–3 mcg/kg IV for induction
Onset	Peak effect 3 min
Offset	10–20 min
Side effects	Respiratory depression, bradycardia, hypotension
	Chest rigidity (high doses)

7.1.2   Alfentanil

This is a synthetic opioid. More rapid onset than Fentanyl.

Indications	Attenuate response to laryngoscopy
Presentation	Clear solution containing 500 mcg/mL (2 mL amp)
Dilution for use	Neat
Dose	20 mcg/kg IV
Onset	Peak effect 90 s
Offset	5–10 min
Side effects	Same as Fentanyl

7.2   Induction Agents

Ketamine and Propofol are probably now the most commonly used induction agents for PRSI within the UK. Ketamine has certainly become the first choice induction agent for trauma patients for both GNAAS and London HEMS.

Ketamine has gained in popularity in recent years encouraged by the number of British military doctors working in UK HEMS who have worked in Afghanistan as part of the Medical Emergency Response Team (MERT). Ketamine was the standard induction agent for PRSI within the MERT from 2008. It was selected as the safest induction agent in young patients who were often hypovolaemic following massive trauma. The beta-1 and alpha-1 effects can help to maintain blood pressure, whereas Propofol (which is the most frequently used induction agent in hospitals in the developed world), causes vasodilation and an element of myocardial depression. Together with the sudden reduction in endogenous catecholamines following anaesthesia, this can cause profound hypotension. Due to its sympathomimetic effect on beta-2 receptors, Ketamine is also particularly useful for induction of patients with severe bronchospasm.

For many years there was a widely held belief that Ketamine increased ICP and was therefore unsuitable for use in patients with head injury. This misconception appears to stem from early studies that reported increased ICP in patients breathing spontaneously; the effect was almost certainly due to an increase in $PaCO_2$ rather than a direct effect of Ketamine. In ventilated patients, Ketamine often *decreases* the ICP (Zeiler et al. 2014). It is unclear whether the N-methyl-D-aspartate (NMDA) receptor antagonist effect of Ketamine is beneficial or not. In some studies on developing animals, higher doses of Ketamine appeared to have a neurotoxic effect, although these effects were prevented by the co-administration of a Gamma-aminobutyric acid (GABA) receptor agonist (this may be another reason for using Midazolam for ongoing sedation following a Ketamine based RSI) (Himmelsher and Durieux 2005).

Overall; the maintenance of blood pressure following induction and a stable or reduced ICP (which results in a stable or increased cerebral perfusion pressure (CPP)) leads to a recommendation to use Ketamine in patients with head injuries requiring PRSI.

In elderly patients who are not shocked, the hypertension and tachycardia following Ketamine may potentially risk myocardial stress and ischaemia, however, with a lower induction dose and pretreatment with Fentanyl, this is probably less of an issue than the potential for hypotension which may result from using Propofol. Tachycardia following Ketamine induction also has the potential to cause some confusion regarding depth of anaesthesia, as both tachycardia and hypertension are usually signs of inadequate anaesthesia. Those who do not routinely using Ketamine in their clinical practice should keep this factor in mind.

Propofol or Thiopentone would normally be the induction agents of choice for a patient with status epilepticus. Ketamine is not recommended in these patients.

Etomidate was previously advocated as the best induction agent for PRSI (EMS Physicians 2006), and was the standard induction agent used by both GNAAS and London HEMS for almost a decade. The benefit of Etomidate is that when compared to most other agents, it is relatively cardiostable. It causes less hypotension than Propofol and Thiopentone, without the tachycardia of Ketamine. Etomidate also reduces ICP and cerebral metabolism. These effects result in a stable CPP and a reduction in cerebral oxygen requirements. This made it a seemingly ideal induction agent for most pre-hospital patients requiring PRSI. Unfortunately it is now clear that Etomidate induces temporary (12–24 h) adrenocortical dysfunction. It has been shown to inhibit 11-beta hydroxylase production of cortisol, leading to decreased serum cortical levels. This is associated with an increased mortality when used in patients with sepsis and may potentially have detrimental effects on trauma patients (Chan et al. 2012; Warner et al. 2009). Combined with the general acceptance that Ketamine does *not* cause an increase in ICP, Etomidate has therefore fallen out of favour.

7.2.1   Ketamine

This is a phencyclidine derivative.

Indications	Induction of anaesthesia in patients with hypotension or asthma
	Potent analgesic; ideal for facilitating extrication
Presentation	Clear colourless solution containing 10, 50, or 100 mg/mL (**Beware using the incorrect concentration**)
Dilution for use	10 mg/mL (e.g. 200 mg made up to 20 mL with 0.9 % NaCl) IV
	50 mg/mL when used IM
Dose	Profound analgesia 0.25–0.5 mg/kg IV (1–4 mg/kg IM)
	IV induction 1–2 mg/kg IV (5–10 mg/kg IM)
Onset	30 s
Offset	5–10 min
Side effects	Emergence phenomenon hallucinations or unpleasant dreams during recovery. Incidence reduced by Midazolam and recovery in a stimuli free environment
	Tachycardia and hypertension
	Relative contraindication in ischaemic heart disease
	Masseter spasm
	Increased salivation
	Increased upper airway reflexes. Instrumentation of the upper airway without muscle relaxant may lead to laryngospasm

7.2.2   Propofol (2,6-Diisopropylphenol)

This is now the most commonly used induction agent in UK hospitals and is also widely used for sedation in critically ill patients.

Indications	Induction and maintenance of general anaesthesia
Presentation	White oil in water emulsion containing 10 mg/mL (1 %) (20 mg/mL (2 %) is also available)
Dilution for use	Neat
Dose	1.5–2.5 mg/kg IV induction (up to 4 mg/kg in Paeds) IV maintenance of sedation at a dose of 2–6 mg/kg/h
Onset	15–20 s
Offset	5–10 min
Side effects	Pain on injection (reduced by adding Lidocaine) Hypotension (particularly in hypovolaemia)

7.2.3 Etomidate

This is a carboxylated imidazole.

Indication	IV induction of anaesthesia
Presentation	Clear colourless solution for injection containing 2 mg/mL
Dilution for use	Neat in a 10 mL syringe
Dose	0.2–0.3 mg/kg
Onset	30 s
Offset	8–10 min
Side effects	Adrenocortical dysfunction Pain on injection (reduced by adding Lidocaine) Myoclonus (abnormal movements)

7.3   Muscle Relaxants

A muscle relaxant with rapid onset is required for PRSI. Suxamethonium is the most rapidly acting muscle relaxant currently available, and its effect wears off within a few minutes in most patients. Some people believe that this property is an advantage in the 'can't intubate, can't ventilate' situation, as the patient may start to breath before critical hypoxia occurs. In reality, this is unlikely to be the case (Benumof et al. 1997). Using Rocuronium and then giving a dose of Sugammadex (16 mg/kg) to reverse the effect will return normal muscular activity far more rapidly. Realistically, this 'wake up' option is rarely a luxury available to the pre-hospital provider of anaesthesia, as the patient would not normally be anaesthetised if it was possible to get them to hospital safely without intubation and ventilation. In the failed intubation scenario it is usually better to use an alternative airway technique (i.e. supraglottic airway) rather than allow the patient to wake up.

Rocuronium is now the relaxant of choice for PRSI; optimal intubating conditions are present 60 s after a 1.2 mg/kg dose providing a speed of onset almost as rapid as Suxamethonium. A Cochrane Database systematic review in 2008 found no statistical difference in intubation conditions when Suxamethonium was compared to 1.2 mg/kg Rocuronium (Perry et al. 2008) Rocuronium has the additional advantages of: rapid reversal with Sugammadex, fewer side effects, and does not require a second drug to be carried to provide ongoing muscle relaxation for transfer.

If Suxamethonium *is* used, a non-depolarising muscle relaxant is normally given following successful intubation to prevent the patient coughing or resisting ventilation during transfer when the effect of Suxamethonium wears off. This is preferable to the alternative option of using higher doses of sedation, which is more likely to result in unwanted hypotension. Vecuronium is probably the non-depolarising muscle relaxant of choice for this purpose as it has a medium duration of action (30–40 min), has a low incidence of anaphylaxis and does not require refrigeration. It does need to be reconstituted with water prior to use. Atracurium is an alternative, but requires refrigeration to avoid degradation. The choice of muscle relaxants used will depend on the team and the system in which they are working. However it should be predetermined in system protocols, and regularly practised by the team members to ensure familiarity.

7.3.1   Rocuronium

This is a non-depolarising muscle relaxant.

Indication	Facilitate intubation and maintain paralysis in an intubated patient
Presentation	Clear colourless solution containing 10 mg/mL
Dilution for use	Neat in a 10 mL syringe
Dose	Intubation 1.2 mg/kg IV
	Supplementary dose 0.15 mg/kg
Ideal intubation	60 s (1.2 mg/kg)
Effect time	20–60 min dependent on dose (0.5 mg/kg or 1 mg/kg)
Side effects	Pain on injection, anaphylaxis (incidence same as suxamethonium but 10 × higher than other relaxants) mild vagolytic

7.3.2   Suxamethonium

This is a depolarising muscle relaxant.

Indications	Rapid onset paralysis as part of RSI
Presentation	Clear colourless solution containing 50 mg/mL (2 mL amp)
Dilution for use	Neat
Dose	1–1.5 mg/kg IV bolus
Ideal intubation	30–40 s

Effect time	3–5 min usually
Side effects	Prolonged action (sux apnoea) in 4 % lasts for 10 min to 2 h
	Fasciculations resulting in muscle pain
	Temporary raised intra ocular/cranial pressure
	Hyperkalaemia (burns and spinal cord injury) *but only >24 h after injury*
	Malignant hyperpyrexia (and masseter spasm)
	Bradycardia
	Anaphylaxis
Notes	Should be stored at 2–8 °C (potency loss 2 %/ month at 21–25 °C)

7.3.3   Vecuronium

This is a non-depolarising muscle relaxant.

Indication	Maintenance of paralysis in an intubated patient
Presentation	Lyophilised powder
Dilution for use	Diluted with 5 mL of water to yield a clear, colourless solution containing 2 mg/mL that is stable for 24 h
Dose	Initial 0.1 mg/kg
	Supplementary dose 0.05 mg/kg
Ideal intubation	3–5 min
Effect time	40 min

7.3.4   Atracurium

This is a non-depolarising muscle relaxant.

Indication	Maintenance of paralysis in an intubated patient
Presentation	Clear colourless solution containing 10 mg/mL (5 mL amp)
Dilution for use	Neat in a 5 mL syringe
Dose	Initial 0.5 mg/kg
	Supplementary dose 0.1–0.2 mg/kg
Ideal intubation	3–5 min
Effect time	25–35 min
Side effects	Histamine release (avoid in asthma)
Notes	Should be stored at 2–8 °C (potency loss 5 %/month at 25 °C)

7.4   Sedation

Several agents can be used to sedate patients. Short acting agents e.g. Propofol, must be given by infusion to avoid large variations in blood pressure. Bolus doses or large changes in infusion rate are not recommended as they can lead to cardiovascular instability. Infusion pumps do, however, require batteries or an external power source and introduce an additional complexity to the handling of patients.

Longer-acting agents e.g. Midazolam can be administered by intermittent bolus dose. Bolus dosing of Midazolam can also lead to hypotension; careful attention should be paid to the blood pressure after each bolus. It is recommended that a small dose should be given initially followed by careful titration depending upon patient response and blood pressure.

Ketamine may also be used for sedation by intermittent bolus, but effects on heart rate, blood pressure and cerebral metabolic rate mentioned earlier must be kept in mind (Box 7.1).

Box 7.1: Aims of Sedation
- Prevent awareness/recall
- Prevent hypertension and tachycardia
- Reduce cerebral oxygen requirement

Adequate sedation may result in hypotension especially in hypovolaemic patients. This effect is predictable and may be managed with a fluid bolus or bolus dose of a vasoactive drug e.g., Ephedrine 3–6 mg. Care should be taken not to 'over treat', as surges of blood pressure may worsen haemorrhage (Box 7.2).

Box 7.2: Factors Influencing the Choice of Sedative Agent
- The familiarity of the individual with sedation technique
- Availability of an infusion pump (ideally required for shorter-acting drugs)
- The cardiovascular status of the patient (avoid Propofol in hypotension and Ketamine in hypertensive patients
- Chronic medical conditions
- The length of transfer (setting up an infusion for a short transfer may be inappropriate)
- The expected clinical course on arrival at definitive care

All individuals administering sedation should be familiar with the indications, dosing regime, contraindications and side effects of the agent used. Continuous vigilance is required for the signs of inadequate sedation (Box 7.3).

Box 7.3: Signs of Inadequate Sedation
- Tachycardia
- Hypertension
- Dilated pupils
- Lacrimation
- Sweating

A mix of Morphine and Midazolam has been recommended for sedation, 10 mg of each can be diluted in the same syringe to 10 mL.

Give 0.05–0.1 mg/kg (e.g. 3.5–7 mL), followed by repeated doses of 0.02 mg/kg (1–2 mL) during transfer, every 10–20 min as indicated. If an infusion device is available the intermittent bolus technique can be replaced by an infusion at an initial rate of 0.1 mg/kg/h.

7.4.1 Midazolam

This is a benzodiazepine.

Indications	Hypnosis and sedation
	Management of emergence phenomenon
	Anticonvulsant
Presentation	Clear colourless solution containing 10 mg in 2 mLs (10 mg in 5 mLs also available)
Dilution for use	1 mg/mL (e.g. 10 mg diluted to 10 mL with 0.9 % NaCl)

Dose	0.05–0.1 mg/kg (lower dose in elderly) initially
	0.02 mg/kg maintenance bolus (1–2 mg in adults)
Onset	1–2 min but can take up to 15 min for maximal effect.
Offset	Variable and dose dependent but can be up to 2 h.
Side effects	Respiratory depression
	Hypotension
Notes	It can be used as an anticonvulsant. For these purposes bolus doses of 0.5–2 mg should be titrated to effect. It may be useful in the management of emergence phenomenon after Ketamine administration but co-administration increases the likelihood of airway compromise.

7.4.2   Morphine

This is an opiate.

Indications	Analgesia
	Combined with Midazolam for sedation
Presentation	Clear colourless solution 10 mg/mL (1 mL amp) (Beware 30 or 60 mg/mL 1 mL amp)
Dilution for use	1 mg/mL
Dose	0.05–0.1 mg/kg initially titrated up to 0.2 mg/kg
Onset	Peak effect IV after 15 min
Offset	2–4 h
Side effects	Respiratory depression, hypotension, urticaria, phlebitis

7.5 Analgesia

7.5.1 *Morphine*

Morphine has long been the gold standard for the relief of severe pain in hospital and also for pre-hospital analgesia in the military. The benefits are that it provides good analgesia and the effect lasts for at least 2 h. The onset of Morphine is relatively quick (a few minutes), however, the peak effect only occurs 15 min after administration. Therefore the potential exists to give repeated doses without waiting for the peak effect of the previous dose. This may result in respiratory depression that could manifest itself during transfer. Morphine is well suited for the provision of analgesia for a constant level of pain but is not ideal for procedural analgesia (e.g. extrication or traction realignment of a fracture) due to the time of onset and then long offset.

7.5.2 *Fentanyl*

Fentanyl is an alternative to Morphine. The onset and peak effect (3 min) is much quicker and this makes it an attractive choice. The effect time is around 20 min, which will provide adequate analgesia for short transfers; however, hospital staff may need to give further analgesia soon after arrival. For longer journeys it is advisable to administer Morphine instead, or in addition to, the initial dose of Fentanyl.

7.5.3 *Entonox*

Entonox is excellent for relief of short periods of extreme pain and is used widely in hospital medicine (e.g., during labour, relocating dislocated joints). The fact that it requires a compliant casualty and is contraindicated in suspected chest injuries limits its use in pre-hospital management of major trauma.

Entonox is a 50:50 mix of nitrous oxide and oxygen. It is administered via a demand valve, so requires adequate respiratory strength and patient compliance. It has a 30 s onset (so the casualty needs to breath the Entonox for 30 s before the painful stimulus) and an offset of only 60 s. Other analgesia is usually required as well, with Entonox used for any short periods of increased pain.

It has minimal cardiovascular, respiratory or neurological effects but is contraindicated when there would be a risk from expanding any gas filled space within the body (i.e. a pneumothorax). This is due to the fact that nitrous oxide will diffuse into the space faster than the nitrogen within the space can diffuse out leading to a build up of pressure.

7.5.4   Ketamine

Ketamine is useful for managing relatively short periods of extreme pain when nitrous oxide is contraindicated or unavailable. It can provide adequate analgesia without loss of consciousness with a dose as small as 20 mg (0.25 mg/kg). Respiratory effort and blood pressure should be maintained during a period when the management of either may be difficult. For these situations it therefore has particular advantages over Fentanyl or Morphine.

Ketamine is the drug of choice to provide dynamic analgesia i.e. analgesia suitable to facilitate intermittent intensely painful procedures. Dissociative anaesthesia occurs at higher doses (1–2 mg/kg). This is a state of dissociation from consciousness and the patient will appear in a trance or fugue state with their eyes open. Airway reflexes and spontaneous respiration are usually preserved. Increased airway secretions and nausea can be a problem. Hallucinations on awakening from anaesthesia can also be an issue. This side effect may be minimised by giving a small dose of Midazolam.

7.5.5   Local Anaesthesia (Appendix "Local Anaesthetic Blocks")

Local anaesthesia can occasionally be useful in the pre-hospital environment. A femoral nerve block can provide excellent analgesia for a femoral shaft fracture. It should ideally be used before applying a traction splint. Digital nerve blocks are simple to perform for dislocated fingers.

The volumes described in Appendix "Local Anaesthetic Blocks" are for adult patients. Children require smaller volumes. Safe doses of local anaesthetics for adults and children are:

Lidocaine	3 mg/kg	(1 % Lidocaine = 10 mg/mL)
Bupivicaine	2 mg/kg	(0.5 % Bupivicaine = 5 mg/mL)

7.6   Cardiovascular Support

7.6.1   Adrenaline (Epinephrine)

This is a catecholamine and acts as an inotrope, chronotrope and vasopressor.

Indications	Anaphylaxis
	Cardiac arrest
	Low cardiac output states
Presentation	Clear solution containing:
	0.1 mg/mL (1:10,000) 10 mL prefilled syringe or 1 mg/mL (1:1,000) 1 mL amp

Dilution for use (and dose)	*1:1,000*–0.5 mL (0.5 mg) IM in anaphylaxis 12 years to adult
	(0.3 mg 6–12 years, 0.15 mg 0–6 years)
	1:10,000–10 mL in cardiac arrest (0.1 mL/kg in children)
	1:100,000–1 mL of 1:10,000 diluted to 10 mL with 0.9 % NaCl. Use 1–2 mL boluses titrated to response in hypotension.
Side effects	Dysrhythmia
	Tachycardia and myocardial ischaemia
	Lactic acidosis

7.6.2   Ephedrine

This is a sympathomimetic amine.

Indication	Hypotension (has an indirect effect – may be relatively ineffective in elderly)
Presentation	Clear colourless solution containing 30 mg/mL (1 mL amp)
	Or 3 mg/mL (10 mL autojet)
Dilution for use	3 mg/mL (one ampoule 30 mg/mL up to 10 mL with 0.9 % NaCl)
Dose	3–6 mg (1–2 mL) titrated to response
Side effects	Unlikely (hypertension and tachycardia)

References

Benumof JL, Dagg R, Benumof R. Critical hemoglobin desaturation will occur before a return to an unparalyzed state following 1 mg/kg intravenous succinylcholine. Anesthesiology. 1997;87:979–82.

Butler J, Jackson R. Lignocaine premedication before rapid sequence induction in head injuries. Emerg Med J. 2002;19:554.

Chan CM, Mitchell AL, Shorr AF. Etomidate is associated with mortality and adrenal insufficiency in sepsis: a meta-analysis. Crit Care Med. 2012;40:2945–53.

Himmelsher S, Durieux ME. Revising the dogma: ketamine for patients with neurological injury? Anesth Analg. 2005;101:524–34.

Lyon RM, Perkins ZB, Chatterjee D, et al. Significant modification of traditional rapid sequence induction improves safety and effectiveness of pre-hospital trauma anaesthesia. Crit Care. 2015;19:134.

National Association of EMS Physicians. Prehosp Emerg Care. 2006;10:260.

Perry JJ, Lee JS, Sillberg VA, Wells GA. Rocuronium versus succinylcholine for rapid sequence induction intubation. Cochrane Database Syst Rev. 2008;(2):CD002788. doi:10.1002/14651858. CD002788.pub2.

Warner KJ, Cuschieri J, Jurkovich GJ, Bulger EM. Single-dose etomidate for rapid sequence intubation may impact outcome after severe injury. J Trauma. 2009;67:45–50.

Zeiler FA, Teitelbaum J, West M, Gillman LM. The ketamine effect on ICP in traumatic brain injury. Neurocrit Care. 2014;21:163–73.

Chapter 8
Special Circumstances

By the end of this chapter you should understand the specific management issues associated with:

- Hypothermia
- Paediatrics
- Obstetrics
- Head injury
- Transferring patients by air

8.1 Hypothermia

This is defined as a core temperature less than 35 °C. It is associated with a number of undesirable effects:

- Cardiovascular arrhythmias occur at 30 °C, ventricular fibrillation (VF) at 28 °C
- Vasoconstriction makes intravenous access difficult and increases myocardial work
- Increased blood viscosity reduces tissue perfusion
- Thrombocytopenia – platelets are sequestered in the liver and spleen
- Shift of oxygen haemoglobin dissociation curve to the left – worsens oxygen delivery to tissues
- Reduced level of consciousness (unconscious at 30 °C)

T. Lowes et al., *Pre-Hospital Anesthesia Handbook*,
DOI 10.1007/978-3-319-23090-0_8,
© Springer-Verlag London 2016

There are two main issues to be dealt with in the hypothermic casualty: dealing with the hypothermia, but also appreciating and managing the reason for the hypothermia. The casualty who has simply become overwhelmed by the cold needs careful handling and possibly intubating (depending on Glasgow Coma Score (GCS)), prior to transportation to a hospital where they can be re-warmed. In severe cases the use of cardiac bypass may allow more rapid warming and transfer to a unit capable of doing this should be considered. Some of these cases may be due to alcohol excess causing reduced consciousness and loss of awareness of cold. It is important to consider that unconsciousness may have preceded hypothermia, e.g. head injury, vascular intracerebral event, hypoglycaemia, severe hypovolaemia etc. Depending on the diagnosis, these patients may be better transferred to a neurosurgical or trauma unit with emphasis on managing the underlying injury rather than rapid warming.

Patients with multiple trauma and no head injury have been shown to have a markedly worse outcome if they are hypothermic. In this patient group a core temperature of <32 °C is invariably fatal (Jurkovich et al. 1987). One reason may be because coagulation depends on enzymes which function best at 37 °C. Hypothermia therefore impairs blood clotting and will potentially result in increased blood loss. Hypothermia may also partly be a marker of the severity of haemorrhagic shock, and the resultant depression of metabolism and heat generation by the body.

It is not usually possible to increase core temperature in the pre-hospital environment. Management should be aimed at minimising further heat loss. This is done by removing wet clothing, sheltering from wind/rain, covering with heat reflective blankets, using heat-generating packs (care must be taken to avoid skin burns) and increasing the ambient temperature of the transport vehicle. The hypothermic patient who has suffered cardiac arrest should be treated as per national guidelines (usually with double the interval between drug dosages and fewer attempts at defibrillation until normothermia is achieved).

It can also be difficult to diagnose death in the hypothermic patient. Unless there are obvious external signs of death (e.g. de-capitation), or a good history of death preceding hypothermia, it is probably best to use the mantra 'they are not dead, until they are warm and dead'. This means keeping resuscitation attempts going until the casualty is in the hospital at the very least.

A meta-analysis of eight randomised controlled trials (RCTs) of therapeutic hypothermia after traumatic brain injury led the Brain Trauma Foundation to issue a Level III recommendation for the optional and cautious use of hypothermia following traumatic brain injury (TBI) in adult patients (Peterson et al. 2008). Good quality evidence is, however, lacking. In 2009 a Cochrane meta-analysis (Sydenham et al. 2009) on 23 trials with a total of 1614 patients found no convincing evidence that hypothermia was beneficial in TBI patients. They selected RCTs of hypothermia to a maximum of 35 °C for at least 12 consecutive hours in patients with closed TBI, and investigated effects on death, Glasgow Outcome Scale and pneumonia. Out of these trials, only nine were of good quality and concealment. Although results showed an overall trend towards benefit for hypothermia to reduce deaths (OR 0.85, 95 % CI 0.68–1.06), significance was only found in the low quality trials. No improvement in mortality was found with the high quality trials (OR 1.11, 95 % CI 0.82–1.51). There are trials ongoing that may help to address this (EUROTHERM 3235 Trial, NABIS: H IIR)

Hypothermia maintained after out of hospital VF cardiac arrest has been accepted therapy in order to improve neurological outcome (European Resuscitation Council 2005). A Cochrane review in 2012 also found benefit in neurological outcome by using induced hypothermia after cardiopulmonary resuscitation (Arrich et al 2012). A more recent trial has, however, cast doubt on the benefits of hypothermia (Nielsen et al 2013). This was a large (939 patients), well-designed RCT, and the results were unequivocally negative. Following this, some editorials have called for therapeutic hypothermia to be abandoned, rather aiming for a temperature of 36 °C and ensuring that *hyper*thermia does not occur, as this is undoubtedly associated with worse outcomes. Others have highlighted potential issues with the trial and believe therapeutic hypothermia should still be used (Stub 2014). The current advice for pre-hospital staff is therefore not to actively rewarm patients who survive cardiac arrest, and that any fever should be cooled if possible.

There is some interest in profound hypothermia (suspended animation) in those trauma patients who arrest when practitioners are present. This, at the moment, can only be described as experimental, and so should be left for controlled research groups.

8.2   Paediatrics

Trauma accounts for up to 40 % of childhood deaths. In a 12 years period London HEMS attended 1933 children (Nevin et al. 2014). There were 315 (16.3 %) pre-hospital intubations; 81 % received a rapid sequence intubation (RSI) and 19 % were intubated without anaesthesia in the setting of near or actual cardiac arrest. The most common injury mechanisms in this population were road traffic incidents and falls from height. Intubation success was 99.7 % with only a single failed intubation during the study period. Eich et al. (2009) reported similar success rates (98.3 %) for pre-hospital paediatric intubation.

There is as yet no evidence to support the assumption that intubation is superior to assisted face mask ventilation for the treatment of children less than 12 years or weighing less than 40 kg in terms of survival or neurological outcome after injury. The only randomised controlled trial is poor quality, looks at non-drug assisted intubation and is inconclusive (Gausche et al. 2000). Many pre-hospital doctors will have limited, if any experience, of anaesthetising children, and as children desaturate much more quickly than adults when they stop breathing, the threshold for pre-hospital anaesthesia (PHA) may be higher than for adults.

If the age of the child is known at dispatch then drug doses can be calculated en-route to the scene. Drug dose calculators and Broselow tapes can help in doing this effectively. Whenever drug doses are calculated for children it is sensible to check the dose with another trained crew-member.

A child is not simply a miniature adult and a more considered approach should therefore be taken when preparing for intubation. The paediatric airway differs significantly from the adult airway (Table 8.1). This may require an alteration in intubation technique.

The airway is smaller and as a result requires increased dexterity for manipulation and specialised equipment. The tissues of the airway are softer and more pliable. This means airway obstruction is more likely at extremes of head position and with relatively little external pressure, especially under the chin when supporting a face mask.

Children have a disproportionately large head relative to their chest until around the age of 8 years old. This forces the cervical spine into relative kyphosis (head flexion) when lying on a firm surface. Young children (<3 years) should

TABLE 8.1 Comparing infant and adult airways

	Infant	Adult
Tongue	Relatively larger	Relatively smaller
Larynx	Opposite second and third cervical vertebrae	Opposite fourth, fifth, and sixth cervical vertebrae
Epiglottis	"U" shaped, large, floppy	Flat, flexible, erect
Hyoid/thyroid separation	Very close	Further apart
Smallest diameter	Cricoid ring	Vocal cord aperture
Consistency of cartilage	Soft	Firm
Shape of head	Pronounced occiput	Flatter occiput

have a 1–2 cm pad under their chest and nothing under their head to provide an optimal intubating position (see Fig. 8.1). To ensure transport with the neck in a neutral position (particularly when there is concern regarding cervical spine injury), children under 9 years old should be transported with a pad/blanket under their chest (Herzenberg et al 1989). The correct thickness of support is best judged by aligning the external auditory meatus with the centre of the shoulder.

In neonates and infants (<1 year) the relatively large size of the tongue may make it more difficult to sweep and displace during the laryngoscopy. Using a curved blade in the vallecula may still leave the "floppy" epiglottis hanging down over the vocal cords obstructing the view. Going behind the epiglottis and lifting it with the tip of the blade is appropriate in these cases. To use this technique a straight-bladed laryngoscope is required to give the optimum view of the larynx.

The arytenoids in infants slant away from the intubator during laryngoscopy. This may prevent the endotracheal tube from passing easily. A 90° anticlockwise rotation usually remedies this. If this is not the case, a smaller size tube maybe required.

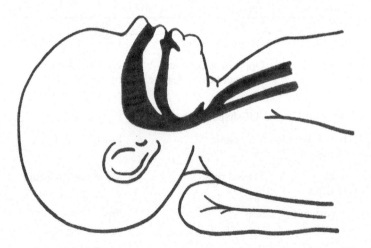

FIGURE 8.1   Chest elevated by blanket for optimal intubating position

The cricoid ring is the narrowest part of the paediatric airway. An endotracheal tube that is too large may pass through the cords, but not the cricoid ring. In these cases a smaller tube should be selected. All manipulations of a paediatric airway must be much gentler than in an adult as the structures are delicate and prone to oedema. An infant's airway is typically 3 mm in diameter. A 1 mm circumferential swelling leaves an airway 1 mm in diameter. This is a 68 % reduction. The same degree of oedema in an adult airway will only reduce the diameter by 25 %.

Uncuffed endotracheal tubes have traditionally been used in children less than 10 years of age. This allows the use of a larger diameter tube minimising airway resistance and maximising airway toilet. It is important to ensure that a leak is present above 15 cm H_2O to prevent excessive pressure on the mucosa. Aspiration is less likely as the cricoid ring has a round aperture that should seal around the endotracheal tube. More recently, cuffed endotracheal tubes have been advocated. They may be beneficial with chest injuries when relatively high ventilation pressures are required.

Endobronchial intubation is relatively common in paediatric intubation due to the shorter trachea. It should be expected and excluded by auscultation. Once a satisfactory position is confirmed, the length at the lips should be noted and the tube firmly secured. Head/neck movement should be avoided as this can cause the tube to move significantly both up and down the trachea, potentially leading to partial extubation or endobronchial intubation.

It is not uncommon for children to have loose teeth especially after trauma. Special attention should be paid to avoid aspiration of teeth during ventilation/intubation.

8.3 Obstetrics

The management of the pregnant trauma patient is emotionally charged, as there are two lives potentially at risk. The preservation of the fetus is completely dependent on the effective assessment and resuscitation of the mother. Optimal management of the pregnant casualty requires an understanding of the physiological and anatomical changes that take place during pregnancy and how they impact upon RSI.

From the first trimester there are marked changes in anatomy and physiology, due the increasing levels of progesterone from the placenta. They are widespread and include:

8.3.1   Airway

Increasing deposition of adipose tissue around the neck and breasts complicated by tissue oedema, may make laryngoscopy and intubation more difficult. The risk of failed intubation for obstetric anaesthesia is 1 in 300 (compared to 1 in 2000 general surgical patients).

Gastric emptying and acidity are not changed by pregnancy. But the difference in pressure between the stomach and lower oesophageal sphincter is reduced. During pregnancy, particularly with the onset of labour, administration of opiates or trauma may lead to an increased risk of reflux and loss of lower oesophageal competence making aspiration more likely.

8.3.2   Breathing

The diaphragm may be displaced cephalad by up to 4 cm at term. This means that greater care should be exercised when performing thoracostomy in order not to cause diaphragmatic injury.

There is a 60 % increase in oxygen demand during pregnancy, and a reduction in functional residual capacity of 20 %, which means that the onset of desaturation, even following pre-oxygenation, is rapid.

A rise in tidal volume of 40 % results in a physiological hyperventilation and resulting arterial partial pressure of carbon dioxide ($PaCO_2$) of 4.0 kPa at term. An end-tidal CO_2

$(ETCO_2)$ of 3.5–4.0 should be the goal to reflect physiological hyperventilation of pregnancy.

8.3.3 Circulation

Aorto-caval compression may occur when the pregnant uterus rests on the aorta or inferior vena cava. This reduces venous return and cardiac output as a result. Utero-placental blood flow is not auto-regulated and so is dependent on uterine blood flow. Even in the absence of maternal hypotension, uterine blood flow may be reduced by the supine position. After the twentieth week of gestation, uterine displacement should always be employed. In hospital this is usually achieved by tilting the operating table 15–30° to the left or placing a wedge under the right buttock. In the trauma patient, the most practical method is usually manual displacement of the uterus; literally pulling the abdomen over to the patient's left side, away from the inferior vena cava (Fig. 8.2). A relative reduction in cardiac output may make the pregnant patient feel nauseated and provoke vomiting, even if the blood pressure is normal - this may also be accompanied by auditory/visual disturbances.

Cardiac output increases by 1–1.5 L/min and blood volume increases by up to 50 % out of proportion with the increase in haemoglobin levels leading to a physiological anaemia. The systolic and diastolic blood pressure falls by 5–15 mmHg during the second trimester and rises to normal levels at term. In the third trimester the resting heart rate increases by 15–20 beats/min. These physiological changes mimic the response to hypovolaemia and may be misleading after trauma. In the presence of hypovolaemic shock, shunting from the uterine and placental beds may occur. A blood loss of up to 1.5 L is therefore possible without any change in maternal physical signs. A fluid challenge should be considered in all pregnant trauma victims, as fetal hypoperfusion may be present despite normal maternal parameters. Permissive hypotension is therefore not recommended.

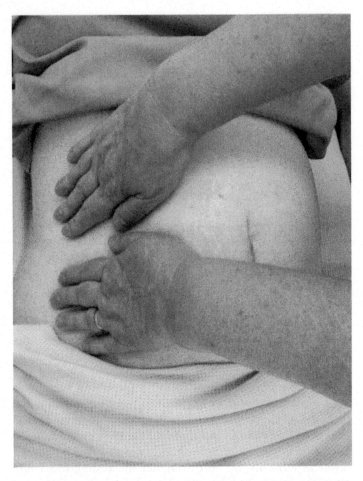

FIGURE 8.2 Manual Displacement of the patient's uterus to the left side

Peripheral vasodilation can make veins more prominent; but the presence of hypovolaemia, increased adipose deposition and oedema can result in difficult intravenous (IV) access.

Pregnant women become hypercoagulable in the first trimester. Plasma concentrations of I, V, VIII, IX, X, and XII are all increased. Antithrombin III levels are depressed. This is the reason for the increased risk of pulmonary embolus in the first trimester.

8.3.4 Disability

If the level of consciousness is altered with no obvious cause, eclampsia (convulsions in pregnancy or following delivery in the absence of other causes) should be considered. Eclampsia almost always occurs in the presence of pre-eclampsia (hypertension, proteinuria and oedema; with epigastric pain and low platelets in severe cases). In these cases Fentanyl should be used to attenuate the sympathetic response to intubation.

8.3.5 Obstetric Referral

It is important to involve an obstetrician as soon as possible when dealing with pregnant trauma patients. Call ahead and alert the receiving hospital before departure. Useful information that should be conveyed includes:

1. Weeks of gestation (fundal height greater than 2 cm above the umbilicus suggests gestation greater than 25 weeks – and may be viable if delivered).
2. Mechanism of injury.
3. Obvious site of injury.
4. Vital signs on arrival and trends over time.
5. Interventions undertaken. If PHA has been undertaken, the drugs given (esp. opiate dose and time) should be communicated as well as the cardiovascular stability during and after intubation.

It should be noted that if a pregnant woman suffers a cardiac arrest, current recommendations are that the fetus should be delivered within 5 min. Every pre-hospital practitioner should have a plan in mind as to how and where this would be best achieved in their area.

8.4   Head Injury

Traumatic brain injury presents a particular challenge in the pre-hospital environment. Injury sustained on impact and prior to the arrival of the medical services is largely irreversible. The aim of management is therefore to avoid secondary injury (Box 8.1).

Box 8.1: Preventing Secondary Brain Injury (Jones et al. 1994)

- The avoidance of hypoxia (PaO_2 >8 kPa or SpO_2 >92 %).
- The avoidance of hypotension (keep Systolic BP >90 mmHg or good volume radial pulse).
- The avoidance of hypo/hypercapnia ($ETCO_2$ of between 4 and 4.5 kPa).
- The avoidance of hypo/hyperglycaemia (4>blood glucose <10 mmol/L).
- The maintenance of normal to high plasma osmolality.

Hypercapnia causes a predictable increase in cerebral blood flow that leads to increased intracranial pressure (ICP). This may have a deleterious effect on outcome in head injured patients with poor intracranial compliance. Conversely, excessive hyperventilation should be avoided because hypocapnia causes cerebral vasoconstriction, which may lead to ischaemia in areas of the brain that have the potential to recover. To avoid this, $ETCO_2$ should be kept between 4 and 4.5 kPa (aiming for a low/normal $PaCO_2$ of 4.5–5.0 kPa). Patients with physical findings suggestive of dangerously high ICP e.g., bradycardia, dilated pupil(s), may be temporarily hyperventilated to prevent coning. The aim for deliberate hyperventilation should be an $ETCO_2$ of 3–3.5 kPa in a stable patient and 2–2.5 kPa in patients with hypovolaemia or chest injury (Helm et al. 2003).

Poor outcome from brain injury is associated with blood glucose levels >10 mmol/L and neurological damage can result from blood glucose levels <1.5 mmol/L. It is possible to manage hypoglycaemia in the pre-hospital environment but it is not recommended to attempt to treat hyperglycaemia. Hyperglycaemia should be treated early on arrival at hospital.

As noted previously the head injured patient *may* benefit from mild hypothermia, and *hyper*thermia should certainly be avoided and treated where possible. Hyperosmolar therapy can be used if raised ICP is suspected (i.e. pupil(s) dilates). There is no evidence of clinical outcome benefit from hypertonic saline over Mannitol; both will reduce ICP. Mannitol (0.25–0.5 g/kg) is effective, however, it may crystallise out of solution in colder climates (rewarming should reverse this). It will also cause a diuresis, which may potentially result in hypovolaemia during longer transfers. In the pre-hospital environment, hypertonic saline is probably a better option (2 mls/kg of 5 % NaCl or equivalent volume of a different concentration).

8.5   Transferring Ventilated Patients by Air

Aeromedical transport of the critically ill patient is a specialty in its own right, however many providers of PHA work out of helicopters. It is therefore important to have a basic understanding of how this mode of transport can affect the patient's physiology.

8.5.1   Altitude

Most pre-hospital evacuation is carried out at altitudes below 2000 m, making the issues of gas expansion and cabin pressure relatively unimportant; however this should still be kept in mind where there is the potential for pneumothorax. For longer transfers (>1 h), particularly at higher altitudes, the endotracheal tube cuff pressure should be monitored to avoid mucosal ischaemia of the trachea.

8.5.2   Temperature

Air temperature decreases with increasing altitude. It is usually possible to control the temperature of the cabin, although this can be more difficult in some helicopters. Increased cabin temperature will only prevent heat loss; it is unlikely to raise the temperature of a hypothermic patient. As for all patients, wet clothing should be removed and heat-reflective/insulating blankets used to retain body heat.

8.5.3   Acceleration/Deceleration

A patient being transferred in a helicopter may experience linear and radial forces. Both these forces may affect cardiovascular stability. Linear forces occur along the long axis of the airframe and a casualty may experience fluid shifts along this axis that may result in hypotension and tachycardia. Radial forces occur due to change in direction and occur outward from the centre of the turn.

Linear forces are particularly significant during take-off and landing in a fixed-wing aircraft. If the patient is positioned with head to the front, take-off may cause a significant period of reduced venous return in a relatively hypovolaemic patient. A dramatic reduction in cardiac output and blood pressure may result. This effect can be reduced by fluid loading prior to take-off. If the patient is positioned feet forward, there will be a period of increased intracranial pressure during take-off that may be detrimental in a patient with traumatic brain injury. On landing the effect is not as pronounced or for as long. Head towards the front and nor-movolaemia is therefore optimal.

8.5.4 Vibration

This is a characteristic feature of helicopter flight. It can lead to blurred vision, shortness of breath, motion sickness and fatigue. It can also interfere with the body's ability to auto-regulate temperature. This is important in heat-related casualties.

Vibration may cause wound disruption, fracture move-ment and bleeding that may lead to increased requirements for analgesia, sedation and resuscitation.

Monitoring vital signs (clinically and by machine) can be impeded by vibration. Taking a pulse can become very diffi-cult and monitors may suffer interference leading to unreli-able data. Newer transport monitors have better software and tend to function better in this environment.

8.5.5 Noise

Listening to a chest is usually impossible in a helicopter due to the noise, so a clinical assessment relies on visual inspec-tion and palpation with reference to airway pressures on the ventilator. It is important to listen to the chest following PHA and before boarding a helicopter, as it is easier (and better) to pick up a developing pneumothorax and deal with it whilst on the ground.

Noise can cause damage to hearing even in unconscious patients and so ear protection should be provided. A spare headset may be available for conscious patients allowing communication during transfer. If not, it is important to explain to the patient that communication will be difficult, prior to leaving. Hand signals may be required to alert the medical team if the patient develops problems en route.

Communication between medical staff and also with the pilot is essential, so all should have linked headsets.

References

Arrich J, Holzer M, Havel C, et al. Hypothermia for neuroprotection in adults after cardiopulmonary resuscitation. Cochrane Database Syst Rev. 2012;(9):CD004128.

Eich C, Roessler M, Nemeth M, et al. Characteristics and outcome of prehospital paediatric tracheal intubation attended by anaesthesia-trained emergency physicians. Resuscitation. 2009;80:1371–7.

European Resuscitation Council. European resuscitation council guidelines for resuscitation 2005. Resuscitation. 2005;67:S1–189.

EUROTHERM 3235 Trial. http://www.eurotherm3235trial.eu/home/index.phtml. Accessed 28 May 2015.

Gausche M, Lewis RJ, Stratton SJ, et al. A prospective randomised study of the effect of out of hospital paediatric endotracheal intubation on survival on neurological outcome. JAMA. 2000;283:783–90.

Helm M, Schuster R, Hauke J, Lampl L. Tight control of pre-hospital ventilation by capnography in major trauma victims. BJA. 2003;90:327–32.

Herzenberg JE, Hensinger RN, Dedrick DK, Phillips WA. Emergency transport and positioning of young children who have an injury of the cervical spine. The standard backboard may be hazardous. J Bone Joint Surg Am. 1989;71:15–22.

Jones PA, Andrews PJD, Midgeley S, et al. Measuring the burden of secondary insults in head injured patients during intensive care. J Neurosurg Anesthesiol. 1994;6:4–14.

Jurkovich GJ, Greiser WB, Luterman A, Curreri PW. Hypothermia in trauma victims. An ominous predictor of survival. J Trauma. 1987;27:1019–24.

Nevin DG, Grenn SJ, Weaver AE, Lockey DJ. An observational study of pre-hospital intubation and anaesthesia in 1933 children attended by a physician-led, pre-hospital trauma service. Resuscitation. 2014;85:189–95.

Nielsen N, Wetterslev J, Cronberg T, et al. Targeted temperature management at 33 °C versus 36 °C after cardiac arrest. N Engl J Med. 2013;369:2197–206.

Peterson K, Carson S, Carney N. Hypothermia treatment for traumatic brain injury: a systematic review and meta-analysis. J Neurotrauma. 2008;25:62–71.

Stub D. Targeted temperature management after cardiac arrest. N Engl J Med. 2014;370:1358.

Sydenham E, Roberts I, Alderson P. Hypothermia for traumatic head injury. Cochrane Database Syst Rev. 2009;(2):CD001048. Accessed 21 May 2015.

Chapter 9
Complications, Adverse Events and Clinical Governance

By the end of this chapter you should:

- Be familiar with the types and incidence of common complications associated with PHA
- Be able to diagnose and manage the common adverse events during transfer

9.1 Complications

All interventions are associated with complications. Understanding the cause of these complications allows the operator to take steps to avoid them and this makes the procedure safer. The incidence of complications during pre-hospital anaesthesia (PHA) is difficult to establish from the current literature. It is likely that the reported absence of benefit from pre-hospital intubation in some studies may result from the complications during and after its performance. One study certainly suggested that an increased mortality was associated with pre-hospital hypotension and hyperventilation in head-injured casualties who underwent pre-hospital intubation (Davis et al. 2004). Other studies have demonstrated that the different make-up of teams and different ways of carrying out the technique make a huge

T. Lowes et al., *Pre-Hospital Anesthesia Handbook*,
DOI 10.1007/978-3-319-23090-0_9,
© Springer-Verlag London 2016

difference – London HEMS report a failed intubation rate of only 0.25 % (Lockey et al. 2013) whilst other systems report rates up to 31 % (Cobas et al. 2009).

9.1.1   Immediate Complications (Box 9.1)

These result from the mechanical technique of laryngoscopy and intubation. Upper airway trauma to the teeth, pharynx, larynx, and trachea results from excessive force or improper use of the laryngoscope blade. This is often compounded when the intubation is difficult or hurried. Prolonged attempts at intubation expose patients to harmful physiological responses and increase the risk of hypoxia and aspiration (Mort 2004). An attempt to intubate should not normally exceed 45 s.

Box 9.1: Cause and Incidence of Immediate Complications	
Complication	**Incidence (%)**
Upper airway trauma to the teeth, pharynx, larynx, trachea (Adnet et al. 1998)	1–5
Failed Intubation (Lockey et al. 2013; Cobas et al. 2009)	0.25–31
Unrecognised Oesophageal intubation (Cobas et al. 2009)	6.4
Endobronchial intubation (Caruana et al. 2015)	16
Adults (Adnet et al. 1998)	2.8
Paediatrics (Easley et al. 2000)	15
Exacerbation of spinal cord injury (with MILS) (Criswell and Parr 1994; Reid et al. 1987)	0

Complication	Incidence (%)
Increased risk of aspiration (Adnet et al. 1998)	5.6–34
Anaphylactic shock (Adnet et al. 1998)	0.3
Bronchospasm (Adnet et al. 1998)	0.8
CVS instability	
Arrhythmias and bradycardia (Mort 2004)	1.6–19
Hypotension (Reid et al. 2004)	17
Cardiac arrest (Adnet et al. 1998)	4
Hypoxia ($SpO_2 < 92\%$)	
Overall (Mort 2004; Caruana et al. 2015; Dunford et al. 2003)	18–57

9.1.2   Early Complications (Box 9.2)

These usually arise during transfer. The complications include endotracheal tube migration leading to accidental extubation or endobronchial or oesophageal intubation. One study reported 12 % of patients on arrival in hospital had unrecognised oesophageal intubations, although this was following non-drug assisted paramedic intubation (Cobas et al. 2009). Twisting of the endotracheal tube (ETT) or excessive cuff inflation pressures may lead to mucosal damage and an increased risk of subsequent tracheal stenosis. It is important to use a sterile endotracheal tube and ensure that it is kept as clean as possible during pre-hospital rapid sequence intubation (PRSI). Pre-hospital intubation is consistently reported as being associated with pneumonia later on in intensive care (von Elm et al. 2009).

Box 9.2: Early Complications

Complication	Incidence (%)
Barotrauma (pneumothorax, surgical emphysema and pneumomediastinum) (Schwartz et al. 1995)	1
Hypercapnia (Helm et al. 2002)	16
Hypocapnia (Helm et al. 2002)	41
Death within 30 min (Schwartz et al. 1995)	3

9.1.3   Late Complications

These complications can arise as result of the severity of a patient's injury or as a result of immediate or early complications during PRSI (Box 9.3).

Box 9.3: Late Complications

Complications	Incidence (%)
Hypoxic brain injury & multiorgan failure from hypoperfusion	Unknown
Pneumonia (Eckert et al. 2004)	
Pre-hospital intubation	35 %
ED intubation	23 %

9.2   Adverse Events

It is difficult to estimate the incidence of adverse events in the anaesthetised patient during transfer to hospital, however it is unlikely to be less than the incidence during transfers within hospitals. Brunsveld-Reinders et al. (2015) reported a prospective study of transfers of critically ill patients from ICU to other hospital departments (typically for diagnostic procedures). One or more incidents were reported in 133 of 503 transfers (26 %). Many of these are relevant to pre-hospital transfer: hypotension, hypoxia, equipment malfunction, hypertension, cannula dislodgement, empty oxygen cylinder etc.

Too many critical incidents are related to human factors (39 %) or equipment failure (61 %) (Beckmann et al. 2004). These should be preventable with better Crew Resource Management (CRM) training and good equipment husbandry. The use of a checklist may also help (Brunsveld-Reinders et al. 2015).

There are two main adverse events that occur during transfer of a critically ill ventilated patient:

1. Hypoxia (low SpO_2)
2. Hypotension

It is important to be able to rapidly recognise and manage the underlying problem causing either of these two events.

9.2.1 Hypoxia (Low SpO_2)

It is essential to have an action plan to manage sudden patient desaturation (Appendix "Actions on Desaturation").

First check whether the saturation probe is on a finger and has a normal trace. It is not uncommon for the probe to be hanging off the finger or on the floor/tucked in the blankets. Reposition the probe whilst continuing the assessment. If the probe is on and working, move straight on to find the problem.

The problem area can be narrowed down by a simple question: "**Is the chest moving up and down**?" If the chest is moving up and down, the problem is in the patient. If the chest is *not* moving up and down, the problem is generally in the equipment (anywhere from the ETT to the oxygen supply).

9.2.1.1   Chest Moving Up and Down (= Problem in the Patient)

A problem in the patient will be due to a cardiac or respiratory issue, again a simple question should be asked: 'Is there a pulse?'

If there is no pulse, then the patient must be treated as per standard cardiac arrest protocols, although if in Pulseless Electrical Activity (PEA) a tension pneumothorax should be ruled out early.

If the pulse is weak then hypotension is likely, resulting in poor lung perfusion and increased ventilation/perfusion mismatch and a reduction in SpO_2 – give fluids ± adrenaline (epinephrine).

If the pulse is normal then there is a *Respiratory Problem*.

Respiratory Problem

Again simple questions will diagnose the problem: 'What is the airway pressure compared to before the problem started?' (look at the airway pressure gauge on the ventilator). It will be either increased or about the same.

If the airway pressure has increased since intubation, look at the chest movement. If there is evidence of diaphragm/abdominal contraction, then the patient is not adequately paralysed and needs more muscle relaxant (this can be confirmed with the capnograph trace). If not, movement needs to be assessed to see if it is symmetrical or not.

If in doubt, get the self-inflating bag out and hand ventilate. This will give you more of a "feel" for the problem and larger tidal volumes can make asymmetrical chest movement more obvious.

If one side is moving better than the other then consider the factors in Box 9.4.

Box 9.4: Issues to Consider if Chest Movement Is Asymmetrical

- ETT in right main bronchus – pull back
- Tension pneumothorax – needle decompression/thoracostomy
- Main bronchus plugged – suction catheter
- Large haemothorax – increase positive end-expiratory pressure (PEEP)

If chest movement is symmetrical consider Box 9.5.

Box 9.5: Issues to Consider if Chest Movement Symmetrical

- Lung contusions – increase PEEP
- Pulmonary oedema – increase PEEP
- Bilateral secretions (unlikely) – suction catheter
- Bronchospasm (occurs immediately after intubation) – use IV Ketamine for sedation

If the Airway pressure is unchanged then the cause is usually worsening lung contusion/haematoma or pulmonary oedema. All that can be done is to increase PEEP. If secretions are present in the ETT, clear with a suction catheter.

9.2.1.2   Chest *Not* Moving Up and Down (= Problem in the Equipment)

If this is the case, then the problem lies somewhere between (and including) the ETT and the oxygen cylinder. Again a simple question should be asked: 'What is the airway pressure compared to just after intubation?' If the chest is not moving, the airway pressure will either by high or low.

If the airway pressure is high, usually it will be due to either an **occlusion or a kink** somewhere in the ventilator tubing or ETT. The ETT should be checked first, including inside the mouth. Paediatric tubes, being smaller and more compliant, are particularly prone to kinking. Ventilator tubing should then be checked from the patient end to the ventilator and the occlusion corrected. It is highly unlikely that lack of chest movement would be associated with high airway pressure for any other reason (Box 9.6)

Box 9.6: Other Rare Issues to Consider if Chest Is Not Moving

Severe bronchospasm may result in no chest movement, but this would usually occur immediately post induction/intubation.

Periarrest tension pneumothorax may also result in no visible chest movement, but this should have been detected before getting to this stage.

If the airway pressure is low (<10 cm H_2O) then the issue is one of **disconnection** or **ventilator failure**.

If the needle on the ventilator is *completely* still, the ventilator has failed. This is usually due to running out of oxygen for gas-driven ventilators (e.g. Oxylog®, ParaPAC™), so immediately change to a new cylinder, ensuring it has been turned on/the valve opened. If the ventilator is turbine driven, the battery may have failed.

If the needle is moving, but at low pressure, then the issue is one of disconnection or extubation. Inspect the tubing, starting at the patient end. Look at the ETT length at the lips to see if it has moved out and look/feel for air/bubbles from the mouth. Any of these would indicate extubation and the need to re-intubate the patient or to replace the ETT with a supraglottic device (this may be preferable if access for intubation is difficult)

If the ETT is secure, check for disconnections all the way from the ETT back along the catheter mount, heat moisture exchange filter (HMEF) and ventilator tubing to where the tubing connects to the ventilator.

If in doubt, get the self-inflating bag out and hand venti-late. Connect directly to the ETT and attach the oxygen tubing to another cylinder with a fir tree connector. This then takes all of the possible problems (other than the ETT) out of the equation.

9.2.2   Hypotension

Hypotension will be caused by one of the following:

1. **Tension pneumothorax**: Always rule this out before assuming blood loss/sedation is the cause. It should be recognised as a potential with chest injuries. The SpO_2 will be dropping and airway pressure increasing on the ventilator. Look for asymmetrical chest movement (one side moving more than the other).
2. **Hypovolaemia/Anaesthesia**: This is the most likely cause but tension pneumothorax and arrhythmia should always be ruled out first. Treat with fluids ± ephedrine or adrenaline (epinephrine) as indicated.
3. **Arrhythmia**: This will be obvious from a quick glance at the ECG on the monitor. Treat as per Advanced Life Support (ALS) protocols.
4. **Severe Bronchospasm**: This may cause 'breath-stacking' if expiratory time is not long enough to allow complete exhalation. Disconnect from the ventilator temporarily to allow lungs to empty. Reconnect with a lower respiratory rate (6–10 bpm) and no PEEP.
5. **Pericardial tamponade**: Consider this particularly after a penetrating wound to the thorax. Treatment is a clamshell thoracotomy, but this is only indicated during transfer if the patient loses their cardiac output altogether. Otherwise call ahead for surgical assistance in the emergency department.

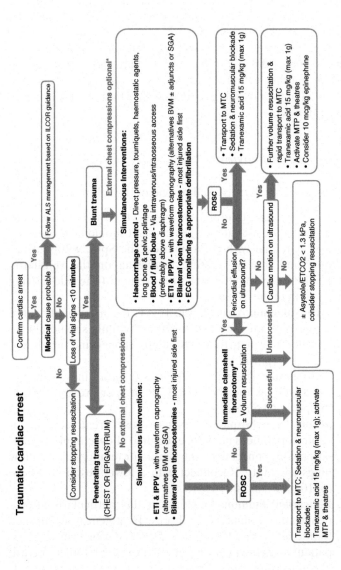

FIGURE 9.1 Traumatic Cardiac Arrest (TCA) and thoracotomy algorithm (Reproduced from Sherren et al. (2013))

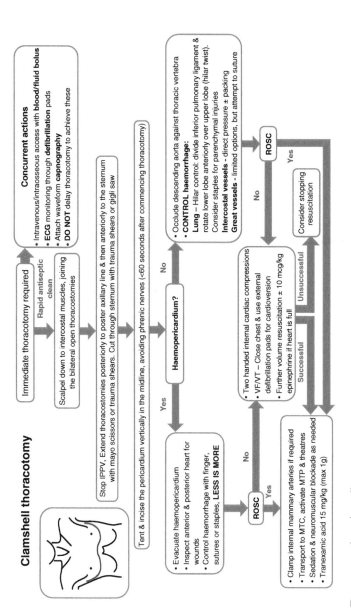

FIGURE 9.1 (continued)

9.2.3   Traumatic Cardiac Arrest (TCA)

If a trauma patient loses cardiac output (i.e. no central pulse palpable) either in your presence or within the 10 min prior to your arrival it is important to rapidly consider and address the potential causes for this in order to maximise the patient's chances of survival. There are three main causes of TCA:

1. Hypoxia
2. Haemorrhage
3. Obstructive Shock (Tension pneumothorax, cardiac tamponade)

Correcting hypoxia is essential as up to 44 % of TCA survivors arrest as a result of asphyxia (Lockey et al. 2006). Intubation and ventilation with 100 % oxygen will address this. This should be followed by immediate bilateral open thoracostomies, which will relieve tension peumothoraces and may reveal evidence of intrathoracic haemorrhage as the cause of TCA. In low velocity penetrating chest or epigastric trauma (e.g. stab wound) this should be extended into a clamshell thoracotomy if there is no immediate return of circulation.

In blunt trauma, the next most likely cause of cardiac arrest is hypovolaemia due to blood loss. Further blood loss must be minimised (tourniquets, pressure/haemostatic dressings, pelvic/long bone splintage) whilst rapid resuscitation (ideally with blood products) is attempted.

External chest compressions are likely to delay all of the procedures described above and may potentially exacerbate injuries and blood loss. For this reason, commencing chest compressions in TCA is not recommended until all of the factors discussed have been addressed.

Sherren et al. (2013) produced a detailed algorithm that describes their approach to TCA (Fig. 9.1).

9.3   Clinical Governance

Regular training and the development and practice of evidence-based (or consensus-based) standard operating procedures (SOPs), should ensure adverse events are kept to a minimum. However, it is inevitable that things will not always run smoothly nor go to plan. When this happens it is important to view it as an opportunity to learn and improve. An open, fair culture enables this learning to take place. Crew debriefing should occur after every task, with any concerns or issues highlighted, and areas for improvement in the future agreed.

Regular confidential case discussion meetings, often known as morbidity and mortality (M&M) meetings, are a feature of many PHA providing organisations. Honest, but non-confrontational discussion is encouraged. Reflection and constructive criticism is expected, whereas derogatory comments and persecution of individuals is not. Mistakes and adverse events should be analysed to identify root causes and system errors, so that preventative measures can be put in place to prevent recurrence. These changes should then make future problems less likely.

Good governance nurtures a safety culture, rather than one of blame. It is important for all members within a pre-hospital organisation to embrace the concept of clinical governance, and for this to be positively led by senior members of staff. Clinical governance is the key to patient safety and improved patient outcomes.

References

Adnet F, et al. Pre-hospital intubation in the French system. Ann Emerg Med. 1998;32:454–9.

Beckmann U, Gillies DM, Berenholtz SM, et al. Incidents relating to the intra-hospital transfer of critically ill patients. Intensive Care Med. 2004;30:1579–85.

Brunsveld-Reinders AH, Arbous MS, Kuiper SG, de Jonge E. A comprehensive method to develop a checklist to increase safety of intra-hospital transport of critically ill patients. Crit Care. 2015;19:214.

Caruana E, Duchateau F, Cornaglia C, et al. Tracheal intubation related complications in the prehospital setting. Emerg Med J. 2015. doi:10.1136/emermed-2013-203372.

Cobas MA, De La Pena MA, Manning R, et al. Prehospital intubations and mortality: a level 1 trauma centre perspective. Anesth Analg. 2009;109:489–93.

Criswell JC, Parr MJA. Airway management in patients with cervical spine injury. Anaesthesia. 1994;49:900–3.

Davis DP, Dunford JV, Poste JC, et al. The impact of hypoxia and hyperventilation on outcome after paramedic rapid sequence intubation of severely head injured patients. J Trauma. 2004;57:1–10.

Dunford JV, Davis DP, Ochs M, et al. Incidence of transient hypoxia and pulse rate reactivity during paramedic rapid sequence intubation. Ann Emerg Med. 2003;42:721–8.

Easley RB, Segeleon JE, Haun SE, Tobias JD. Prospective study of airway management of children requiring endotracheal intubation before admission to PICU. Crit Care Med. 2000;28:2058–63.

Eckert MJ, Davis KA, Reed RL, et al. Urgent airways after trauma: who gets pneumonia? J Trauma. 2004;57:750–5.

Helm M, Hauke J, Lampl LA. Prospective study of the quality of pre-hospital emergency ventilation in patients with severe head injury. BJA. 2002;88:345–9.

Lockey D, Crewdson K, Davies G. Traumatic cardiac arrest: who are the survivors? Ann Emerg Med. 2006;48:240–4.

Lockey DJ, Avery P, Harris T, et al. A prospective study of physician prehospital anaesthesia in trauma patients: oesophageal intubation, gross airway contamination and the 'quick look' airway assessment. BMC Anesthesiol. 2013;13:21.

Mort TC. Emergency tracheal intubation: complications associated with repeated laryngoscopic attempts. Anaesth Analg. 2004;99:607–13.

Reid C, Chan L, Tweeddale M. The who, what and where of rapid sequence intubation. EMJ. 2004;21:296–301.

Reid DC, Henderson R, Saboe L, et al. Etiology and clinical course of missed spinal fractures. J Trauma. 1987;27:980–6.

Schwartz DE, Matthay MA, Cohen NH. Death and other complications from emergency airway management in critically ill adults. Anaesthesiology. 1995;82:367–76.

Sherren PB, Reid C, Habig K, Burns BJ. Algorith for the resuscitation of traumatic cardiac arrest patients in a physician-staffed helicopter emergency medical service. Crit Care. 2013;17:308.

Von Elm E, Schoettker P, Henzi I, et al. Pre-hospital tracheal intubation in patients with traumatic brain injury: systematic review of current evidence. Br J Anaesth. 2009;103:371–86.

Appendices

Appendix A: Pre-hospital Rapid Sequence Intubation (PRSI) Checklist

T. Lowes et al., *Pre-Hospital Anesthesia Handbook*,
DOI 10.1007/978-3-319-23090-0,
© Springer-Verlag London 2016

GNAAS PRSI CHECKLIST

PREOXYGENATION – 02 MASK – BVM – O_2 AND O_2 BACKUP

CANNULA – IN SITU AND PATENT

FLUIDS AND GIVING SET – 500ML CONNECTED AND READY

SUCTION UNIT – WORKING AND BACK UP

MONITOR – ON AND CONNECTED

VENTILATOR – WORKING – SET

DRUGS

      FENTANYL   DOSE CHOSEN

      INDUCTION AGENT   DOSE CHOSEN

      ROCURONIUM   DOSE CHOSEN

      MAINTENANCE DRUGS

IV FLUSH

AIRWAY ADJUNCTS – OPA + 2 NPA

LARYNGOSCOPES – 2 BLADE SIZES – WORKING

BOUGIE

ET TUBES – SIZE CHOSEN (CUFF CHECKED) + SIZE SMALLER

10 ML SYRINGE

CATHETER MOUNT

HMEF

TUBE TAPE OR TIE

CAPNOGRAPH – AND FILTERLINE – WORKING

STETHOSCOPE

IGEL – SIZE CHOSEN

EMERGENCY CRICOTHYROIDOTOMY KIT – AVAILABLE

BASELINE OBS – RECORDED

DRUGS ADMINISTRATOR – BRIEFED

INLINE IMMOBILISER – BRIEFED & C–COLLAR OPEN/REMOVED

CRICOID ADMINISTRATOR – BRIEFED

INJURIES ADDRESSED – HAEMORRHAGE – PELVIC #?

PREPARE FOR TRANSFER – SCOOP, BLANKET, VEHICLE

Appendix B: Drug Dose, Weight and ETT Size Field Guide

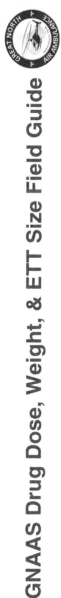

GNAAS Drug Dose, Weight, & ETT Size Field Guide

Drugs	Dilution	Dose
Adrenaline	1 ml of 1:10,000 up to 10 ml with 0.9% NaCl (10mcg/ml)	1-2 ml IV boluses titrated to response
Ephedrine	1 ml (30 mg) up to 10 ml with 0.9% NaCl (3mg/ml)	1-2 ml IV boluses titrated to response
Fentanyl	Neat into 5 ml syringe (50 mcg/ml)	1-3 mcg/kg IV
Ketamine	Neat (200 mg/20 ml) in 20 ml syringe or 4 ml (50 mg/ml) to 20 ml with 0.9% NaCl (10mg/ml) [Use neat neat 50mg/ml for IM]	Analgesia 0.25-0.5 mg/kg IV [1-4 mg/kg IM] Anaesthesia 1-2 mg/kg IV [5-10 mg/kg IM]
Midazolam	2 ml (10 mg) up to 10 ml with 0.9% NaCl (1 mg/ml)	Initial 0.05-0.1 mg/kg IV (lower in elderly) Maintenance 0.02 mg/kg IV (~1-2ml)
Morphine	1 ml (10 mg) up to 10 ml with 0.9% NaCl (1 mg/ml)	Initial 0.05-0.1 mg/kg IV (lower in elderly) Maintenance 0.02 mg/kg IV (~1-2ml)
Propofol	Neat into 20 ml syringe for induction (1%=10 mg/ml) [50 ml syringe for infusion]	Induction 1.5-2.5 mg/kg IV (up to 4 mg/kg in Paediatrics) [2-6 mg/kg/hour IVI. Start ~15 ml/h]
Rocuronium	Neat into 10 ml syringe (10 mg/ml)	1.2 mg/kg IV

Paediatric Weight Calculations (APLS)

< 1 year	(Age in months x 0.5) + 4
1 – 5 year	(Age x 2) + 8
6 – 12 year	(Age x 3) + 7

ETT Size (ID mm)

Adult Male	8.0 mm
Adult Female	7.0 mm
Paediatric	(age/4) + 4 [neonate = 3.0 mm]

ETT Length at teeth (cm)

Adult Male	22 – 24 cm
Adult Female	20 – 22 cm
Paediatric	(age/2) + 12 [neonate = 10 cm]

Appendix C: Failed Intubation Protocol

GNAAS Failed Intubation Protocol

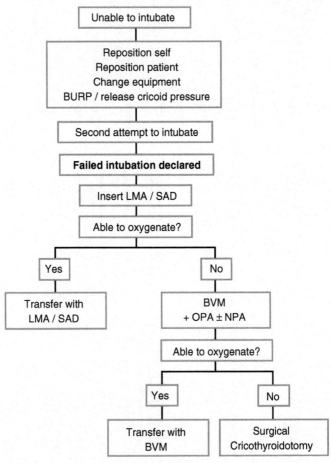

Appendix D: Actions on Desaturation

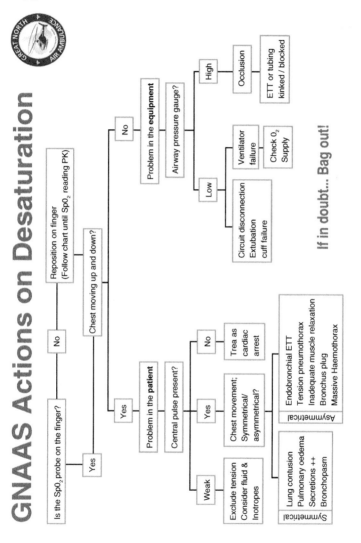

Appendix E: Emergency Cricothyroidotomy

Cricothyroidotomy is an emergency procedure and is usually performed when a secure airway needs to be achieved, and attempts at intubation have failed. It is contraindicated if other less radical means of managing the airway are possible. There is the potential for significant complications, however, it may be a life-saving procedure and the pre-hospital medical team should be trained and prepared to undertake this if required.

The technique of surgical cricothyroidotomy we advocate is rapid, reliable and relatively easy. It addresses two problems that we have commonly seen in the pre-hospital environment which make some of the "standard" techniques less appropriate. These are bleeding from the incision and loss of the track into the airway before or during tube insertion.

Indications

1. Failed airway by all other means.
2. Primary airway under local anaesthetic when PRSI is contraindicated (abnormal anatomy or airway swelling/distortion)

It is a rescue technique for failed intubation in most circumstances. Suitable equipment should be close at hand whenever PRSI is undertaken; this should be included in the PRSI checklist.

In the 'cannot intubate, cannot ventilate situation', cricothyroidotomy is immediately indicated.

Anatomy

The cricothyroid membrane is identified by locating the thyroid cartilage (Adam's apple), and running a finger down the midline until it drops into the cricothyroid membrane

(Fig. A.1). The membrane is bounded inferiorly by the firm cricoid ring. This location is used as it is superficial and has less overlying thyroid and soft tissue than lower approaches. This leads to a lower incidence of significant bleeding.

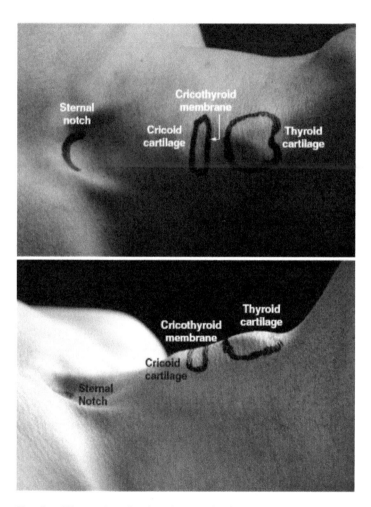

FIG. A.1 The surface landmarks required to perform a cricothyroidotomy

Equipment

- Solution for skin preparation.
- Swabs.
- Short rounded scalpel blade (e.g. No. 15).
- Tracheal dilator/Tracheal hook or small forceps
- Size **6.0 mm** cuffed tracheostomy tube with introducer (or ETT with bougie)
- A 10 mL syringe for cuff inflation.
- Bag-valve-mask (BVM) connected to an oxygen source.
- Securing tapes.

Technique (The Whole Procedure Should Only Take around 30 s)

Different techniques are described in the literature, with no one method demonstrated to be superior. It is important for the PHA team to have one rehearsed technique for prompt management of this critical situation.

1. Prepare all necessary equipment. Ensure the tracheal tube cuff is fully deflated.
2. Hyperextend the neck (a pad/blanket under the shoulders and nothing under the head). During failed intubation this can be assisted by the person attempting to BVM.
3. Clean the skin.
4. Stand/kneel to the side of the patient (usually the same side of the patient as your dominant hand). Immobilise the larynx between the thumb and middle finger of your non-dominant hand. This allows the cricothyroid membrane to be palpated with the index finger.
5. Anaesthetise the skin over the membrane using 1 % Lidocaine if the patient is conscious.
6. Make a transverse puncture straight through the skin and cricothyroid membrane into the trachea. A rounded size 15 blade should ensure this does not perforate the posterior wall. Extend the incision towards you, then

rotate the blade 180 degrees and extend the incision away from you. The incision should be approximately 2 cm long. In cases where excessive soft tissue swelling (oedema, surgical emphysema) makes identification of the cricothyroid membrane difficult, a midline vertical incision of the skin and soft tissues may be performed prior to the transverse incision. A vertical incision is not advocated normally as it adds another stage to the procedure and is likely to cut through one of the branches of the superior thyroid artery as it crosses the midline, resulting in increased bleeding.

7. Insert tracheal dilators/tracheal hook/forceps into the incision alongside the blade *and then* remove the blade.

8. Open dilators/lift the hook/open the forceps and insert the tracheal tube (with introducer inside) into the trachea (some clinicians prefer to use a bougie first and then rail-road the tube over this; this may be useful if an ETT is used, however, this adds an additional stage and the open end of the tracheal tube can catch on the cricoid cartilage as it has to be inserted without the bullet shaped introducer).

9. Remove the tracheal tube introducer and initially confirm the tube position by a quick compression of the chest whilst listening for air expired via the tube. Final confirmation is by gently ventilating with a BVM and seeing end tidal carbon dioxide ($ETCO_2$) on the monitor.

10. Ventilate via the usual catheter mount with heat and moisture exchange filter (HMEF) if paralysed and sedated. If alert with no respiratory failure, a standard oxygen mask may be placed over the tube having attached an HMEF to the tube (to prevent inhalation of dust, etc.).

11. Confirm bilateral chest movement clinically to ensure endobronchial intubation has not taken place if using an orotracheal tube rather than a tracheostomy tube (consider cutting the tube shorter). Fix the tube securely in position with cotton tape or a tracheal tube tie.

12. Suction the trachea if required to clear any blood post-procedure.

Appendix F: Use of Supraglottic Airway Devices (SAD)

Introduction

The Laryngeal Mask Airway (LMA) (Fig. A.2), and further generations of supraglottic devices such as Proseal ™ LMA and i-gel®, are important tools in stepwise pre-hospital airway management.

In position they provide a reasonable seal around the laryngeal inlet, enabling ventilation, and affording some protection to the lungs from contamination by upper airway bleeding. The Proseal ™ (Fig. A.3) and i-gel® (Fig. A.4), also contain a gastric drainage port at the tip of the mask, which sits in the upper oesophagus, allowing free drainage or suction of gastric content, to reduce aspiration risk from gastric contents.

Indications

- To facilitate positive pressure ventilation, when facemask ventilation is difficult or ineffective, despite using simple airway adjuncts and BVM. This may be prior to intubation, or utilised when unable to attempt intubation.
- As a rescue technique for failed intubation.

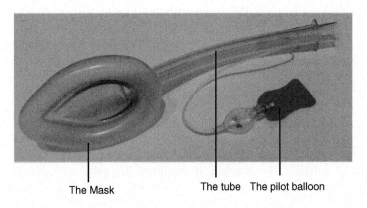

The Mask   The tube   The pilot balloon

Fig. A.2 A laryngeal mask airway (LMA)

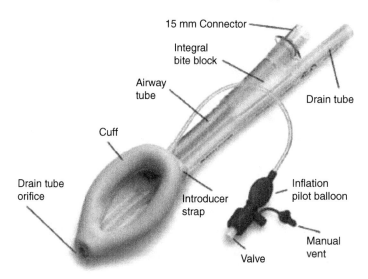

FIG. A.3 A Proseal™ LMA. Reproduced by kind permission of the Laryngeal Mask Company Ltd

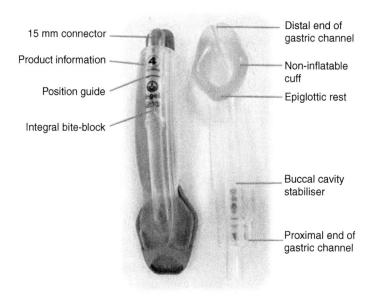

FIG. A.4 I-Gel® supraglottic airway

Equipment

- Appropriate size of device (see Box. A.1).
- Syringe of appropriate volume for LMA/Proseal ™ LMA cuff inflation (this is not required for i-gel®).
- Water soluble lubricant.
- Ventilation equipment (including $ETCO_2$).
- Tie or tape to secure SAD.

Box. A.1   LMA sizes and cuff volumes. (Note; While sized similarly, different devices vary. Such information is displayed on individual devices/packaging)

LMA size	Appropriate patient for use	Maximum cuff inflation volume (mL)
1	Under 5 kg	4
1.5	5–10 kg	7
2	10–20 kg	10
2.5	20–30 kg	14
3	Small adult	20
4	Adult	30
5	Large adult	40

Technique

1. Visually inspect the device, check the cuff (if applicable) in inflation and deflation, leaving the cuff partially or completely deflated in a shape that will easily pass around the tongue.
2. Lubricate the external surfaces of the mask, with water-soluble lubricant. (avoid excessive amounts of lubricant on the anterior surface of the cuff or in the bowl of the mask. Inhalation of the lubricant following placement may result in coughing or obstruction)

3. Extend the head and flex the neck as for intubation, unless cervical spine injury suspected

4. Grasp the device by the tube, holding it like a pen as near as possible to the mask end. Place the tip of the LMA against the inner surface of the patient's upper teeth.

5. Advance the mask along the hard palate, into the pharynx, avoiding the tongue. A jaw thrust by an assistant, or 45° rotation of the device may ease its passage over the tongue.

6. Continue insertion until the device meets with resistance.

7. Inflate the cuff with the recommended volume of air. Often the LMA will rise up slightly out of the hypopharynx as it is inflated and finds its correct position.

8. Connect the device to a self-inflating bag and confirm $ETCO_2$ and bilateral breath sounds.

9. For devices without an integral bite-block, a gauze roll may be placed between the teeth to prevent occlusion of the tube should the patient bite down (this is not required if a muscle relaxant has been used and paralysis is maintained).

10. The SAD can be secured using the same techniques as those employed to secure an endotracheal tube.

Appendix G: Needle Thoracocentesis

This is a potentially life-saving technique for a patient with a suspected tension pneumothorax.

Procedure

1. Find the second intercostal space in the midclavicular line. One method is to identify the manubriosternal joint (angle of Louis). In most people this is a bony prominence approximately 5 cm below the sternal notch adjacent to the second rib. The second intercostal space lies between the second and third ribs. In practice, because of the overlying muscles, this is the first easily definable space you come to on feeling down from the clavicle.
2. Attach a 12 or 14G cannula to a 5 mL syringe. Fill the syringe with 1–2 mL of air or 0.9 % NaCl. After appropriate skin cleansing, pierce the skin and direct the needle just above the third rib (to avoid the neurovascular bundle and reduce the risk of haematoma and intercostal nerve damage). Use a two-handed technique; with one hand supporting the needle by resting against the patient's chest and the other aspirating as the needle is advanced. Upon puncturing the pleura, aspiration of air will confirm the diagnosis (the plunger may be forced out by the high intrapleural pressure). If no air is aspirated, expel the 2 mL of air/NaCl and try aspirating again (there may be a skin plug in the cannula).
3. On aspirating air, stop and advance the plastic cannula, then withdraw the needle. The cannula should be stabilised and secured to prevent kinking or dislodgement.
4. If no air is aspirated, consider the depth of the chest wall and length of the cannula. In patients with large pectoral muscles, it may be necessary to decompress a tension pneumothorax in the fifth intercostal space, just behind the anterior axillary line.

5. Despite initial successful decompression, a cannula may move slightly and no longer penetrate the pleura, and hence cease to function. Be prepared to insert another cannula if signs of tension pneumothorax recur.
6. If the patient is being transported awake, a chest drain must be inserted prior to transfer. If PHA is being undertaken, a thoracostomy must be performed. Positive pressure ventilation can rapidly turn a pneumothorax into a tension pneumothorax or cause reaccumulation of a tension already relieved.

Appendix H: Thoracostomy ± Chest Drain Insertion

Vascular access must be obtained and vital signs monitored. Intravenous fluids must be prepared and ready to give.

Equipment for a Thoracostomy and Chest Drain insertion

- Solution for skin preparation*.
- Sterile gloves*.
- Sterile drape.
- 20 mL syringe and needle.
- Lidocaine 1 % (20 mL).
- Scalpel*.
- Blunt-nosed forceps (e.g. Spencer Wells forceps)*.
- Chest drainage kit including chest drain (e.g. size 28 Fr for adult), tubing and drainage bag with one-way valve.
- Suture material (e.g. 1–0 silk on a hand needle).
- Swabs.
- Scissors.
- Occlusive dressing

(Thoracostomy without chest drain insertion requires only items marked *)

Procedure

Thoracostomy

1. Determine the insertion site. The optimum position is in the fifth intercostal space just behind the anterior axillary line (i.e., just behind the lateral edge of pectoralis major muscle). This is approximately in line with the nipple in the male. Alternatively, count down from the second interspace.
2. Clean the skin (and drape if inserting chest drain).

3. Anaesthetise the skin, intercostal muscles and pleura using 1 % Lidocaine in the conscious patient.
4. Make a 2.5 cm incision through skin and subcutaneous tissue onto underlying muscle. Bluntly dissect apart the intercostal muscles using forceps.
5. Work over the top of the sixth rib to minimise damage to the neurovascular bundle.
6. Puncture the parietal pleura, open the forceps and insert a finger into the incision. Perform a 360° finger sweep to clear possible adhesions between lung and chest wall and exclude any herniated abdominal organs.

In the patient receiving positive pressure ventilation, thoracostomy without chest drain insertion is sufficient to allow drainage of pneumothorax or haemothorax. This avoids the time required to insert and secure a chest drain, as well as the complications associated with performing the procedure in an environment where asepsis is difficult to achieve. A gloved finger may be inserted to reopen the thoracostomy in transit, should there be concern of occlusion and developing tension.

Chest Drain Insertion

7. Attach the tube to the drainage bag. Advance the tube into the pleural space, using the forceps or blunt introducer to aid rigidity. Direct it anteriorly and towards the apex to relieve a pneumothorax (drainage of haemothorax ideally should be left until the patient is in hospital).
8. The tube should be inserted to a distance of 12–13 cm, with all of the side holes of the tube well within the chest.
9. Suture the tube in place, and apply a dressing. Using a 'flag' of zinc oxide tape around the tube and suturing through this is a quick and effective technique compared to traditional 'Roman sandal' methods.
10. Intermittent fogging of the chest tube during respiratory movements, with passage of air or blood into the drainage bag, indicate correct placement. Be vigilant for displacement or blockage throughout transfer.

Complications of Chest Tube Insertion

- Incorrect tube position inside or outside the pleural cavity.
- Laceration or puncture of thoracic or abdominal organs; this can be prevented by the finger sweep before inserting the chest tube.
- Damage to the intercostal neurovascular bundle.
- Dislodgement of the chest tube or disconnection from the drainage bag. Leaking drainage bag. Chest tube kinking or becoming blocked with blood clot.
- Infection (e.g., local cellulitis, thoracic empyema).
- Persistent pneumothorax from large primary defect; a second chest tube may be required.
- Surgical emphysema (usually at tube site).

Appendix I: Local Anaesthetic Blocks

A number of regional anaesthetic techniques can be utilised in the pre-hospital environment, to provide excellent analgesia and reduce the requirement for procedural sedation for fracture reduction. Although ultrasound use is increasing in pre-hospital medicine, local anaesthetic blocks achieved using anatomical landmark techniques without requirement for specialist needles and equipment, are useful to know. An example of such is the Fascia Iliacus block.

Femoral Nerve Block (Fascia Iliacus)

Indication

Analgesia for femoral shaft fractures.

Procedure

1. Clean the skin.
2. Insert a blunted 18G needle just through the skin, 1 cm below the inguinal ligament (runs from anterior superior iliac spine to pubic tubercle) at the junction of outer and middle third.
3. "Pop" through two distinct layers: Fascia lata then fascia iliacus
4. Aspirate the syringe before injecting to check the artery has not been punctured.
5. Inject 30–40 mL of a mixture of 1 % Lidocaine and 0.5 % Bupivicaine.

Onset: 5–15 min.
Duration: Up to 12 h.

Index